ELECTRIC

by

Joshua Holmes

JAHbookdesign | York, PA

ISBN: 9798305243208
Imprint: Independently published

AUTHOR'S NOTE

For veteran and new readers of my books, I wrote four novellas–*Grand Mal, Seizure, Status,* and *Trigger*–comprising The Grand Mal Series, many years ago now, about life with Epilepsy. A lot of it is real, even as I integrated some fiction elements to add levity.

I am compiling them all and republishing them as a multi-part novel called *Electric*. The idea of merging four separate stories into one, offering a collective, intrigued me. I was due to release a book, and I was thrilled with the cover design that emerged. I hope you enjoy!

GRAND MAL
A NOVELLA

JOSHUA HOLMES

PART ONE:

YEAR ONE, SUMMER SEMESTER, SEASONS PAST

THE BUS stop is about ten feet away, near a large ditch, and I plan to sit on a bench until the bus arrives. I have a spot on the bench with my name on it. Chris is my name, and I intend to enjoy a grand summer day, a day with no painful events. The possibility is about to turn unlikely.

I am walking, looking at the golf course just across the way. The green is beautiful, the light turf against the dark rough a vivid landscape, the trees an added accent. The sun is high above in a cloudless sky, and people are riding around in golf carts with their clubs in the back rack. I am walking in a haze. Not a dark haze; a bright haze, if anything. I see the beauty, but I also see more. I see through it, feel a deeper sense of my surroundings. The sense is in my eyes, and in the back of my mouth, an unwanted view and a foul taste. I hope the deeper sense goes away.

I have been walking in this haze for most of the day. I have been living life as I normally would, but I have been carrying a heavy burden, the burden of disastrous possibilities. The possibilities of what may result from these strange sensations, this haze. I just have a small hope my day will continue without interruption.

The sense stays, however, and all of the sudden, it happens. The next thing I know, my body is twisting. My head slowly turns in the right direction, and it continues until my right shoulder rotates in the same direction. My chest is next, and, before I know it, I am falling. A long, hard fall.

I hope someone is near the bus stop, but it doesn't appear there is. If someone was there, I could say, "I'm not feeling good, I need help." Or something along those lines. To my chagrin, however, I don't get the opportunity.

Shortly after, I am on the ground, a road I think. Shaking. Not the kind of shaking most people experience when they are cold or when they have seen something frightening. I mean uncontrollable physical shaking.

I slide towards the ditch that has no business being there. It is right against the pavement. My face digs into the surface. I have faced many surfaces, both indoors and outdoors, yet I still haven't grown accustomed to the burn from my chin rubbing against gravel as black as night, or my forehead attaching itself like a stray weed with strong roots.

GRAND MAL

Strangely enough, I feel no pain when my body suffers. I know it will be bad when I get myself under control. When that happens, if it ever happens, my facial wounds will scream with intensity unlike any other; and my head will pound like a massive wave capsizing a sleepy town. Akin to a punctured ship, my body gradually sinks to the ground.

Upon impact, I bounce off the ground, and roll downward. I am aware of this, because I feel as if I am sliding on an angle. I try to stop rolling, but I am unsuccessful in my attempts. I try to position my body so I won't hit a solid protrusion, whatever it might be.

Soon, though, I am in a deep ditch with no enclaves or rocks to grab onto. Despite my best efforts to avoid injury, I hit something hard, as if I am a swimmer entangled in coral. The walls are too steep. I grapple, but the pebbles just loosen and crumble under my fingertips. I grapple and grapple some more, but the smaller stones start to slide down the wall. I stop momentarily, physically spent. Inside me though, a subconscious force urges me to keep trying. I subconsciously listen.

I hear a voice above me. It says, "I think he fell in the ditch. Over here."

"Yeah, he did," another voice sounds. "I see some foot tracks." Had I seen through some people? I am almost certain no one was around me.

"I'm gonna go check if he's alright."

It feels as if I have been in this ditch for quite some time now. I am sweating profusely, my shirt wet. Maybe it is starting to rain. I don't know. I think I'm starting to go delirious. I look up and ask for this to be over. It's wishful thinking.

The shadows along the walls are lengthy and grey. It was sunny earlier, I know, but there has been a lapse of light since I fell. Darkness covers me now. Gloom, too. Perhaps my current situation has exacerbated my perceptions. It's hard to say.

I groan, struggling to pull myself upright. I try to prop myself up against the dirt wall next to the bench near the bus stop, but I fail. When I hit the bottom of the ditch, most of my body stopped working.

The voices I heard earlier now have faces. Above me, I see two sets of eyes. They all feel sinister. Their stare is penetrating. I see two evil open mouths gawking. They are close to invading my space; an unwanted space, yet my own. I am close to feeling violated. I already have to fight the surface, my own dead body. Now I might have to fight for an open area with no one near.

At one point, I could have hollered for help. Not anymore. When I fell, that was the moment my ability to speak escaped me. I can't even spit out the granules of dirt that have taken my teeth and gum line captive. This is the way it is every time. Inside my throat I am screaming, but no sound escapes my lips. *Just stay away*, I think. *Leave me alone!*

Rarely, though, do people opt to leave me be. The next thing I know, I see an extended arm, and a pointing finger above me. "Should we call the police?"

"Probably. Do you have a cell?" *Shoot!* I think.

• • •

ELECTRIC

I'VE LEARNED to make those who discover me feel better through witticism. If I can laugh about my body contortions, my tremors, my laborious heaving, it appears to make others consider my abnormalities unimportant and something not worth getting upset over. I like it this way, yet I'll never know what they truly feel.

"So, I had the shakes, huh?" I question with a smile.

My friend Michael says, "Yeah Chris. Probably the worst in a while." He acts as if it's no big deal, the response I always hope for. "It's over though. Back to the good life?"

I look at him. He still has a baby face, as round as when I first met him. He has red hair, grizzle on his cheeks, now, and a red goatee. He is well built, also more muscular than I am. He is more outgoing, and quicker to hang with everyone, which explains his reputation as a fun loving guy.

He wasn't always the social butterfly though, the initiator of conversation. In fact, while he was the first to brave my malady, and step out and protect me during a seizure when we were in grade school, he was quite apprehensive to talk. He grew up in a conservative, religious home where it was evil to speak unless spoken to, to have colored hair, tattoos, or piercings for that matter. This mentality branched out into every other area of his life, ultimately forcing him to refrain from any commentary. But he wanted to speak, and eventually became sick of the legalism. He grew weary of hearing "or else you are going to hell."

Whenever Michael did something a little rebellious and heard the threat as a teen, he would say, "Whatever. Back to the good life."

JOSHUA HOLMES

So, kind of joking, I say, "Right. Back to the good life." Truthfully, though, my brain is in a state of turmoil, incredible tides of pain lap on my head of sand.

Michael and I live in a two-room apartment. We split a bathroom, share a small but suitable kitchen, and often recline on the couches in our condensed living room. We agreed I could decorate the living room with my artwork, and he could practice his culinary skills any way he wished in the kitchen. The agreement seems to have worked thus far.

In a short-sleeved Polo shirt and long Cargo shorts, he is standing by the window, a floor to ceiling frame of glass through which you can see the bus stop. "I saw you fall down there," he says, his one hand rubbing his goatee, his other hand in his pocket. "They really need to fill in that ditch."

Michael and I have been friends for years, since adolescence. When we finished high school, we both decided to go to Penn State University, so we wouldn't have to face the postsecondary academic world alone. It has turned out to be a good decision, because, despite the size of this university, we never felt too overwhelmed, and at this point, at ages twenty-five and twenty-six, we find it far from daunting.

I walk over to the window. It is getting dark outside. "Yeah." I say, "That's for sure."

• • •

STILL AT the window, I think of one thing I initially had difficulty with. My ability to communicate with my professors. I found the task irritating, because, in general, my academic success in the Counselor Education program ultimately hinges on the opinions of my superiors. This might be a surprise, but, in the past, I have had several run-ins with one professor. Mrs. Patterson. At times, we just haven't clicked.

I remember one instance when I went to her office to voice an annoyance. The office was as white as snow, spotless, very organized, very little clutter. As with almost every other office in the Rehabilitation Counseling Department, Mrs. Patterson's office had that one seat especially for the student. I eyed the brown chair with plastic armrests, a little wary for I didn't know if I should walk out of the office or proceed with my appointment.

I am always wary of the seat. I think the seat can be inviting if you are making a five-minute, hi and bye visit, but the same seat can be dangerous if you intend to inquire about a professor's reasoning for a poor grade or written criticism for more than ten minutes.

But, being the inexperienced, first year graduate student I am, I decided to question Mrs. Patterson. I never had a chance.

"I just think my grade is unfair," I said. "I made some small grammatical errors, but not enough to warrant a C+!"

"Are you telling me I'm mistaken?" Mrs. Patterson raised her eyebrow, her bright eyes boring into me. I wanted to say she was wrong, that everyone can be wrong at some point.

"I just think it is unfair, because overall, I wrote a good paper!" I became defensive, crossed my arms. "I need a better grade! Please!"

She leaned back in her chair, her hair bouncing as she tipped. "I warned you about the APA guidelines. Plagiarism is unacceptable." I didn't like that accusatory response. It made me feel small, as if I wasn't good enough.

"Chris," she said more sensitively. "Do you understand I gave you the grade because you need practice and can do better?"

I scowled at her, looked down at her immaculate desk. Inside, I knew I was going to blow up. I can't handle it when people don't acknowledge my hard work. "Screw the APA! Screw this! This whole conversation is pointless!"

Again in a softer tone, she said, "I'm sorry, Chris. But I'm not going to change my mind."

"Whatever."

That response got me nowhere. I learned shutting up was the best way to get by. My experience helped me empathize with Michael, as I now have to hold my tongue in my department. Since the meeting, though, Mrs. Patterson and I have learned to agree to disagree. I still hate the APA (American Psychological Association) writing format, and I still have my theory on the chair, but I have refined my communication style.

• • •

As MICHAEL and I walk away from the window and to the middle of the room to settle down, I conclude my concerns about communication and relationships, among other issues relating to my seizures, are almost nonexistent when my mind is elsewhere. Knowing this, I remember, at the start of the school year, Michael and I purchased a wide-screen television to clear our heads when necessary. We split the cost down the middle so it wouldn't empty our

ELECTRIC

pockets, and we often watch it at night in the living room. We will tonight. I don't know about Michael, but I need to ease my feelings of tension.

Of course, studying is priority. Unfortunately. I can't empty my head until I have read, studied, or worked on papers for a while. Michael and I situate ourselves on the floor, and we begin deliberating over our assignments in silence. I always work hard, but I don't necessarily enjoy my efforts. I want to be carefree. Especially tonight, for my seizure has taken its toll.

I have seen Michael, on the other hand, works hard, and loves doing so. Even now. He will lie on his stomach and read and write with great interest, totally absorbed. I take the same position on the cheap carpeting and do the same thing, but whatever I read leaves my mind instantly. Clearly, Michael is a better student.

He has a pen behind his one ear always, and two highlighters behind his other. When he sees a valuable piece of information, he quotes a phrase for which he is known. "Hmmmm. Interesting." He then slides a highlighter from beneath his tuft of hair and marks the page. His Dad was a strong advocate of highlighting notable work when growing up, very strict about regiment. Often, his other highlighter will slide out of position, and fall to the ground. This annoys Michael, but I think it's funny and laugh anyway. He keeps on highlighting, and I can't help but admire his work ethic.

Tonight, a bag of Fritos separates us both, the smell of salty tortilla chips lingering in the air. We share the addictive treat; eat the whole bag usually. Despite the grease on my fingers, I type on my laptop. I skim my material for important quotes, and then reword them on my pc. I hate silence, and keep looking at my watch. When our hour is up, I think, *Thank God!*

Michael keeps reading but he speaks up. "You know, I haven't hosted my debate club in a while. I want to start up again." Michael is a very analytical person, and he likes to voice his opinions in a healthy setting. He listens to others share their stance, and then respectfully sorts through inconsistencies in their views, ultimately questioning its validity. His ability amazes me.

Perhaps the constant barrage of oppressive, religious reprimands at home impacted him so radically he thought it was better to question solid truths and embrace the unknown. He says no, but because I'm a counselor in training, I recognize the influence of atmosphere on a person transitioning into adulthood. In my opinion, this is basic stuff.

I ask him, "Wouldn't you rather join a club that considers the plausibility of multiple factors supporting a view? It would be much more positive that way." I have suggested this before, and he prefers to continue in his pessimism; just like some professors I know. Always in an acceptable environment, he emphasizes with a laugh. "It's fun!" he says. I smile, shaking my head. I'm not going to argue with him.

"Anyway . . . You ready for some Monday night football?" I ask. "Steelers are playing I think."

"Yeah. I think you're right." I quickly walk to my room, and return with my yellow, terrible towel.

GRAND MAL

"Go Pittsburgh." Michael says, putting his pen, highlighters, and books away, and pulling out the little black and gold foam football we throw around during the game.

Although he has retired, I cautiously yell, "Bettis all the way, baby!" Still recovering from my seizure, I don't feel like my normal self quite yet, and I don't want my excitement to induce any undue pain. Let me tell you, though, there is nothing like a good game on the tube to dull a headache, and clear my mind.

• • •

AFTER WATCHING television this night, I get in bed for some well-deserved relaxation. My mattress cradles me like a mother does her baby, and my head rests comfortably on a pillow of cotton clouds. I am a light sleeper and a heavy dreamer, and I hope to sleep well.

Before I fall asleep though, my mind starts to pace back and forth in a hall of memories. As it paces, it recalls times in my life, most of them upsetting. These times are upsetting because I didn't ask for them. I received unwanted attention for a condition I wish didn't exist. My condition, seizure activity as a result of Epilepsy, made me a focal point, a focal point that forced upon me more pressure to please, dependence, and initiated resentment towards others who expected gratitude for their so-called help.

Due to the disturbing nature of my condition, like many with disability-related impairments, I usually provoke confusion, apprehension, and ultimately fear in others. Except for Michael. Even in the most upsetting circumstances, at fourteen years old in seventh grade, he never lost his composure. He kindly pushed everyone else away, and laid my sweaty head in his lap.

I remember a girl named Mary Grace, a nice girl a year younger than us, who sat down next to Michael when he waited for me to come back to life. She always whispered, "It's all right Chris. Everything will be alright." If anyone else had said that, I would have been irritated beyond words, but she was angelic. She was all a boy could want, had blue eyes, long blond curly hair, a white dress, and a halo in my mind's eye. At the time, I didn't know her that well, but I knew she was a caring person who was not concerned with being popular, who had good grades, and who could become a good friend. "He will be alright," Michael always assured her, confidently rubbing his chin.

Looking back, despite having a faithful friend in Michael, and a supportive girl in Mary Grace, I worried constantly I would lose them and any future friends as a result of my seizures. I was different. I am still different. I had no way of telling whether the kids would avoid me because I could potentially interrupt their free time, and I'm not sure anyone would acknowledge this concern even today.

Persons, places, or events that make me worried, angry, or sad haunt me in various ways when I dream, and hypothetical possibilities emerge in rapid succession until I stop trying to sleep. A few of the biggest instigators of these dreams are the loss of friendship, rejection, and humiliation.

On these nights when my mind races, I do eventually tell myself, even though there haven't been many, I have had friends, and my mind slows to a jog.

ELECTRIC

• • •

A DAY AFTER my seizure, and an hour before lunch, I gather my materials and jog downtown to Starbucks for a flavored Chai tea. Inside, I hear Louie Armstrong on the radio, singing 'What a Wonderful World', one of my all-time favorites. Louie's raspy voice makes me feel light-hearted. I sit down and listen to the bluesy tune for a minute, then pull out my laptop. Usually, I play games on my computer, my preference either arcade or sports-related. I must be a funny sight, because I wince every time I lose or die. I do try to keep myself under control, but sometimes I could hop from my chair and scream out of frustration.

All about me, students are sitting at small tables, and have their hands wrapped around their mugs of coffee or tea. Some are studying. Some are talking with friends. Others are just thinking, casually passing away time. I am casually passing away time, too. Maybe not productively, however.

I am resorting to computer games instead of social and physical activities. For years now, I've settled for cartoons jumping and racing on a screen at my command as opposed to doing so myself, as opposed to participating in an activity with others. I could get too anxious or too overwhelmed, I've always thought, potentially causing a seizure.

I kind of want to take a risk though. Before my surgery, I did get involved in karate, and my seizure level decreased a great deal. I have frequently thought about the times I went to my karate class, and how good it made me feel. I want to have that feeling again.

JOSHUA HOLMES

And I can. Just down the street, on the way here, I saw a gym sign advertising a free karate lesson, and despite the safety precautions by which I should abide, I decide to check it out, to see if I can fight.

• • •

IT IS a fight getting through the door at Starbucks, but I make it outside, where students and faculty are chatting at round tables under green, Starbucks umbrellas. From there, I head to a busy place outdoors, art supplies in hand. I then sit under the summer sun with my pencil and drawing pad, to sketch people as they walk beneath the canopies of branches and leaves that hang from oaks all around.

Today, in particular, I sit on one of the benches that face the steps of Old Main, a beautiful building with a cobblestone exterior, several windows with cream-colored window frames, and a large steeple. Many group rallies are held here, so the surrounding courtyard is normally congested with people. For hours, I try to compose a portrait as I listen to the sounds of campus life, the university bell chime, the singing birds, the student conversations and laughter.

These days remind me how important drawing is to me. It is a form of therapy that alleviates my angst, and a release that allows me to express myself in a very personal way. When I was young, I enjoyed sharing my love for creativity with Michael, and he loved watching me.

We'd lay in my back yard, under a large tree with damaged bark. He would lay on his back, hands behind his head, resting in the soft soil, and look up at the oak's wooden fingers as I lay on my stomach, scanning my surroundings for an inspirational piece of nature to put on paper. Once I found what I wanted, I would run my idea by Michael, and he would either approve or make helpful suggestions.

As a beginning artist, I was a big fan of color experimentation. I still am. For a time, however, I worked with one main color. Michael was supportive of my artistic liberties, as well.

Back then, my seizures impacted my drawing style a great deal. During my teenage years, my seizures were accompanied by repeated nightmares of being shackled to a weight, falling in a never-ending whirlpool of clear blue water inside a gothic church. I would be submerged in liquid, drowning, gravity's death grip tugging from the depths. I would see stray Bibles and hymnals float on by me as I was sucked into a bottomless abyss of dark blues. With all the shades of blue in these dreams, I started using excess amounts of the color in my drawings. I remember Michael pushing his red hair out of his face, dirt caked on his forehead, and commenting on my change in style.

"You know, Chris, your drawings are much different than they used to be."

"It's just like in my seizures, Michael," I would say. "Really blue. Almost Van Gogh blue."

Michael didn't have an artistic eye, and still doesn't. However, when I was drawing in shades of blue that day, he sat up and said, "I'm gonna try to draw you a picture." I was thrilled he wanted to participate in my activity, so I gave him my pad to work on. Before I knew it, he had drawn an abstract looking girl with a halo above her head. He smiled. "I saw the way you were looking at Mary Grace in class today. Now you can look at her all day."

We laughed together a lot. Laughing with my only real friend, a rare but good memory. Outside Old Main again, I have an epiphany. I now know what I'll put on paper. I see a tall girl with curly blond ringlets in a white dress walk up the steps. The bell chimes as she reaches the last step and I press the tip of my pencil to the piece of paper.

• • •

WALKING ON Pollock Road, still thinking about the times I used blue in my art, I notice the blue tint of the sky isn't as bright as it was when I started drawing. White cumulus clouds have moved in, hiding much of the color. What a marvel, nature is.

Looking at the clouds consume the sky, slowly moving ahead, something else occurs to me. I haven't seen my doctor forever. Huh. Well how does my mind go from blue pastel work to nature to my doctor, you ask? The pills I take are blue. It's almost too ironic.

I'm on three medications, actually, but I'm not certain how effective the blue pill, Depakote ER, is. I would like to speak with my neurologist about other options. While I do not entirely trust him, I make a mental note to give the doctor a call when I get home.

First though, under the cover of clouds, I am going to go to the HUB.

• • •

ON A regular basis, I go to the HUB Robeson building, the center of activity, where all the undergraduates usually mingle. All the

ELECTRIC

restaurants on the ground floor, Italian, Chinese, and fast food, are available to the students for most of the day. I prefer the fast food.

It is important for me to be around the hustle and bustle, the fast paced routine of academic life. Otherwise, I waste time in my room, bored to tears because I don't know what to do with myself. Despite the constant flow of kids who meander haphazardly, and the loiterers in the lobby, I find the HUB the most relaxing place on campus.

It is a three-tiered structure. I usually sit in the lounge area on the first floor, below the second and third floor offices. Several green chairs are set sporadically so students and teachers who are tired can rest, eat, watch news on the big screen television, or use the hot spots to work on their laptops, allowing them to finish up assignments. I bring my laptop with me, and cross my fingers in hopes of a free electric socket for my charger.

It's not surprising I have to write a lot of papers. After all, I am in graduate school. It is nice to have a place like the HUB to type up grants and summaries of specific research styles.

When I'm not doing this, however, I find a chair hidden behind one of the artificial planters, and I close my eyes and reflect.

I think about the bumpy roller coaster I rode at age nine, the wind rustling my hair with its gusty hands, the bumps, twists, and turns on the tracks that caused the return of my seizures. After five years of normalcy, of perfect physical health, I convulsed violently after the ride. My family and I were devastated.

We had planned to spend a relaxing day at an amusement park, which we did; we watched caricature artists make funny pictures of people, we ate hotdogs and various sweets provided by street vendors, and we played games, my favorite being ski ball because the clown laughed at me when I missed the holes. We never thought, though, a wooden construct meant to entertain would bring our fun to a halt, and cause me any harm. This occurrence preceded years of hospital visits.

The lounge area is normally relaxing, but today it is getting claustrophobic. To my left, an older gentlemen has opened the school newspaper, *The Daily Collegian*, to glance at the weekly editorials, a girl to my right is curled up in a fetal position sleeping, and right in front of me, a young man is playing with a new iPod, his headphones blaring. I really need to go. There is a Barnes & Noble bookstore in the basement of the HUB, thank God. So I shut down my laptop, and walk towards the stairs that lead there. It is busy in the basement too, I know, but there are books. My favorite.

• • •

BEFORE I even get to the stairs, though, I see some of Michael's colleagues. I can tell they are checking out a girl, because they are whistling, then nudging each other in the ribs, and then laughing with one another, still stealing glances at her as she walks ahead of them.

I think, *No wonder women think men are pigs. But, you know, who can blame us? There are so many beauties at this university!* I steal a few glances myself, but am interrupted when the guys approach me, yelling out, "Hey! Chris!"

I say, "Hey guys. What's goin' on?"

GRAND MAL

John, Michael's good friend, says, "So Chris, we were gonna go to the Deli this weekend. You open to coming? Michael said he was." He shifts on his feet, as antsy as a toddler. I've heard he always has to move about. And I think I recall Michael telling me he was like a real Forrest Gump growing up, always running from bullies, which makes sense.

If I remember correctly, John's mother was a teacher, and when any of his peers earned a bad grade, a day in detention, or a visit to the principal's office, he took the brunt. He was in a rough spot, resents his mother for it, I think, and it is, unfortunately, very apparent today. His nerves are fried.

"That would be great." I smile, thinking, *Hmmm. Wow. Someone actually wants me to be a part of something.*

John taps his feet on the floor, obviously eager to reply. "We'll have to give Michael a hard time about the girl he's been talking to."

"He's interested in this girl?" I question, shocked.

"Oh yeah." He laughs, instigating laughs from Alex, one of the other guys making a scene.

Alex is an overweight fellow with beady eyes, a stubby nose, and rosy cheeks. His receding hairline reveals numerous creases in his forehead. When picking on others, he bursts with hilarity, and his creases fissure like uneven ground during an earthquake. His forehead moves back and forth when he asks, "You didn't know?"

I don't like the tone in Alex's voice and I'm about to say something sarcastic about his weight, but I hold my tongue. Michael also told me not to be offended by Alex's behavior. I guess, growing up, he didn't know his parents, jumped from foster home to foster home, his only relatives his grandparents, both of whom made fun of him. Unfortunately, while Alex resented his grandparents, he learned from them the art of verbal abuse, and uses it to make himself feel better. Good old human nature for you.

I find it so interesting how people adjust behaviors to adversities in life, and continue to maintain the same behaviors after the hardships have ended. Whereas John ran away from his problems and developed nervous habits, Alex confronted his adversaries by belittling them.

I don't respond to Alex's question but I bet there are a few creases on my forehead. I turn to leave. Close by, at the information desk, a ticket sales person from the Bryce Jordan Center is distributing tickets to as many students as possible, to clear the long line preventing me from moving. Perhaps *Hairspray*, the Broadway musical, has come to town. Musicals seem to be popular here at Penn State.

As I continue to make my way downstairs, I am still awestruck by the fact I didn't know about Michael's love life. It is big news to me.

• • •

INSIDE BARNES & Noble, I pass the girl at the cash register, the selection of school materials, the frame display, the assortment of officially licensed hats, sweatshirts, sweatpants, and more, and go to the shelf holding all the new nonfiction novels.

Ironically, I find a black book about a person with a disability, an inspirational sort. The inside of the cover gives a brief synopsis of a blind man who climbs a mountain, his difficulties and successes, a real dynamic tale.

ELECTRIC

I stand here quietly in my Penn State paraphernalia, trying to avoid nearby shoppers, and flip through the beginning pages, skimming over the preface and reading the prologue. It is a story that captures my attention, and I want to buy it. No money, unfortunately. It inspires me, though, to tell my story. I sure haven't climbed a mountain, but I have lived through a big setback.

The seizures led to a one-month stay in the neurology department at John Hopkins hospital. I remember the smell of disinfectant, of alcohol, and bad hospital food. I remember smelling of sweat because I didn't bathe daily, and of iodine at times.

I recall the small size of the hospital room, how most of my family and visitors had to stand when they came to see me. Yes, there were chairs, but very few, forcing visitors to take turns if they wanted to sit. There was a small TV bolted to one yellow, concrete wall for their entertainment, but with all the nurses checking on me, no one could really enjoy a movie or show. There was a window that made the room feel a little more open.

I remember lying in the motorized hospital bed, cold, bare, and vulnerable, my skin as white as the anesthesiologist's latex gloves. In my little hospital dress, making sure the IV in my arm didn't get in the way, I tried to conceal myself under the green blankets.

In my most vulnerable state, I met my friend Michael. He was in the room across the hall from me, and he was almost ready to leave the hospital for good, only a week to go. His surgery was successful. No more medicines needed, no more special diets, no more seizures.

JOSHUA HOLMES

Sometimes when Michael and I sit in the living room of our apartment now, I ask him why he thinks his surgery was successful, and why mine was not. We haven't yet come to a reasonable conclusion.

We both have the same scars marking our heads, and we both share traumatic memories, but his life improved, and mine took a turn for the worse. In the end, we agree my circumstances could be the basis for the universal question of why bad things happen to good people.

I recollect the first day I was permitted to leave the hospital room, in a wheelchair pushed by one of my parents or grandparents, all of whom took turns staying with me. I saw Michael in the corridor with his Mom, who happened to be carrying a King James Version Bible. One of the accompanying nurses waved Michael in my direction and introduced him to me shortly after.

"I hope your surgery helps you Chris," I remember Michael saying after we hung out for a week, becoming immediate friends. "I really do."

With no fear, or absolute naivety, I said, "I hope so, too."

"When you get out, maybe we can play." That thought made me happy. And that's how our bond originated. We traded addresses and promised to stay in touch. He left shortly after, and I wrote him daily until medical procedures occupied most of my time.

In the next couple of weeks, I went through several painful tests, medicinal experiments, and long meetings with the surgeons. I was excited at times. I was unsure at times. But mostly, I was miserable.

Before I went into the surgery room very early in the morning on "the big day", my head was shaven clean but free of any hurt.

GRAND MAL

When I was rolling down the hall, I said to my parents, "God will be with me." And He was and is. But He allowed a great deal of suffering. When I came out of surgery twelve hours later, my head was wrapped in a turban, as if I had been born in the Middle East. The wrapping held my skull together, knotted so tight the firm cloth hammered nails of pain above and behind my tender ears.

I was warned there was a possibility I might die under the knife. My parents and I took the risk, signing the contract. Obviously, I am still here. I fought the fight, reading, writing, and drawing to take my mind off of my hospital stay.

I read a book then, and I am reading a book now. The blind mountain climber survived, and so have I.

• • •

WHEN I arrive at the Deli, I don't have the book about the mountain climber on me, but I see a menu I can peruse. Michael is on his way. John, Alex, and some other guys I don't know are already here. They are sitting at a booth nearby, so I bypass the customers in line, grab the menu, and look at it as I head to where they are. I am eager to learn more of the girl Michael is talking to, and curious to see how Michael will respond to the jabs his colleagues will most likely inflict, all in good fun of course.

To be honest, I'm just glad I'm at this restaurant. In my opinion, it is the best culinary establishment in State College. The Deli is a part bar, part formal restaurant. It satisfies both the frequent student customers, and the occasional, visiting parents. The food is just great, and the flavored, Hawaiian tea is unlike any you will find in town.

JOSHUA HOLMES

I am hungry, so I say hello to everyone, sit down, call over the waitress, and order the Deli's classic potato soup. The guys are laughing, nudging each other, and staring at a girl again, another waitress, as she walks into the kitchen. She has a smirk on her face, too.

John says, "She's a looker, huh Chris?" I smile, sort of embarrassed.

"Yeah." I say softly, trying not to let her hear. "She's pretty." They all chuckle at my response. Especially Alex. He adds, "True. True," a comment I'd later learn he adds to every response he gives.

"Glad you came," John says. "Wanted you to be here to celebrate Michael's find." John is a small guy, very comparable to myself, actually. But a similar stature is all we have in common. Whereas I have a goatee and a thick head of dark brown hair, John's face is bare, and his head is totally bald.

"Me too." I say. "It's always fun to be with friends." Inside, I am still wondering why Michael hasn't told me. I then look around, and I reconsider whether this place should be classified as formal, or more pop-culture. It can be both, really. The tables have candles in the center, and the napkins are shaped like fans, but on the walls, a big golden bull head is mounted, a picture of Betty Boop covers a large space, and objects like sleds, coke bottles, and barber shop signs hang, almost placing me back in the Norman Rockwell era. I really wouldn't look all that out of place here if I read the old *Saturday Evening Post*.

Michael arrives when my potato soup comes out. I couldn't have planned it better myself. He grabs a chair from another table, and sits at the head of the four-top. "Hmmm. Very interesting crew, here."

ELECTRIC

"True. True," Alex says, his fat thumbs pointing upwards. "How's the new love of your life, Mikey?"

"She's fine," Michael says. "It's nothing serious, yet."

"Yet?" John replies, laughing and stomping his feet on the ground. "Yet? Did you hear that guys? There's a yet!" They all give each other high fives. I offer a high five, even though I'm not excited like the rest of them.

Michael blushes, goes red in the face. "Honestly. Just hanging out with her for now."

"Hanging out with her where?" John asks, insinuating something I don't even want to think of.

"Yeah! Where?" the rest of them chime in. The jabbing continues, and Michael gets redder and redder. I enjoy myself, but then I remember I have other things to accomplish. So, I finish my soup, and get up.

"Gotta go, guys. Had fun." I say, giving handshakes to them all. I have a hard time fitting my hand around Alex's stubby fingers. Poor kid. "I've got a paper due in my psychosocial class tomorrow."

• • •

AFTER I finish my paper, sitting on an uncomfortable, wooden chair before my desktop computer, I pick up my phone from its cradle, my fingers sore from typing, and punch in the number to my doctor's office. I know he has gone home for the day, and probably is not on call, but I intend to leave a message.

Outside my nearby window, I see it is starting to rain. The white sidewalk leading to the front entrance of my apartment gradually turns a shade of gray as the once dry concrete pads soak up the water droplets. The parking lot is filling up too, each pothole in the pavement overflowing. It is a good night to be inside.

I listen to the phone ring until an answering machine picks up. It takes a while, but I eventually hear the recorded voice of my doctor's secretary ask me to be specific with my information. I begin speaking after the beep.

"Hello, this is Chris. Just wanted to talk to the doctor about my seizures, and to see if he will help me in adjusting my dosage, or changing it all together. Thanks." I relay my phone number and time I should be in.

The wind rattles the walls of my room, and the rain picks up speed. It is so relaxing.

• • •

ON THE days I have my psychosocial class, I have to take the red and white CATA bus from my apartment to the campus. The ride is short, maybe five minutes. However, at times, depending how full the bus is, it feels longer. The transportation service is great, but I don't think CATA considers the comfort of their customers.

On a more positive note, while many of the drivers lack enthusiasm, they are timely. I punctually arrive at the first on-campus stop, at the Patee-Paterno library. The library towers over me. Four beige light posts make the front doors highly visible, and a pine green, life-size abstract gives an ultra-modern effect. The lilacs in the nearby stone planters emit a fresh scent. I marvel at Joe Pa-

GRAND MAL

terno's generosity, for donating so much money to improve the overall quality of the structure.

I observe the students as they stand under the concrete columns that support the square overhang. They read or smoke when they aren't studying inside, and hide from the rain if they are waiting on a ride. I then walk to the Counselor Education building. I travel on foot about five minutes, pass the Chambers building, the brick College of Education sign wrapped in mulch and flowers, and then follow the sidewalk to the CEDAR building entrance. As I make this daily walk I think about my irritating transportation predicament. I've always had the predicament.

Because of my seizure disorder, I have never had the opportunity to drive. I never experienced the excitement of driving a car on my sixteenth birthday. I was so envious of Michael because he was able to do what I couldn't, own a car. To have to ask others to take me places was and continues to be awful, dark thoughts of this fact claw at my psyche. As you might have noticed, I am already a passive person, an introvert who thinks about things that trouble me. An inability to take myself to certain places by myself is a constant reminder of what able-bodied people can do on a regular basis, and of what I cannot. When I have to depend on another person's wheels, I feel like a burden.

In middle school, if friends or family members promised to take me places, and they changed their minds, or circumstances arose that disrupted the plans, I would be ticked. My anger would then turn to sadness. *Why does this always happen to me?* I would think. I also feared upsetting my family members and friends because I didn't know how my responses would affect my daily plans. My plans could be ruined by a look, a facial expression, a reluctant word. It is still a worry.

No time to worry now though. It is time to work. Once inside the CEDAR building, I walk up three flights of stairs to the top floor, and delve into a long white corridor where offices with closed wooden doors on either side conceal the professors within. My class is in a conference room at the end of the hall, just beyond the offices. I take in a deep breath and blow out, preparing myself for a three-hour discussion on disability.

• • •

I HAVE TO admit talking about disability culture in general feels strange to me since I do have a condition that places me within this particular culture. Unlike some with my disorder, I don't like acknowledging the accompanying stigma, much less accepting it for what it is. Why make an issue out of it?

"Disability culture is such an important issue in our field." My professor, Miss Love, reminds me. "After all, we as counselors have to understand psychosocial aspects, how our client will respond to us, and what makes them respond the way they do."

I look around the conference room. It is a small room, all white except for a few flyers taped to the wall advertising Chi Sigma Iota (honor society) events. In the center, my colleagues and I sit around a glossy, mahogany table with our text and notebooks in front of us. There are eleven of us, all of whom are unique and different, sarcastic and fun, but also analytical and critical thinkers.

ELECTRIC

In hopes of not being called on again, I say, "I agree." And I leave it at that.

Talking for three hours can be tedious. Normally, I participate so I learn more, keeping in mind it will pass the time more quickly as well, but this topic is not one of my favorites, so I drift off.

I think about what really contributed to my perceived place in society. Yes, I had seizures before adolescence, but my hospital visits and eventual brain surgery really sealed the deal. The types of seizures and new intensity of the brain activity after surgery changed my life. Looking back, it was about power. I think it's safe to say power is involved in every person's place in society, but when it comes to my disability, my seizures, and the doctors and surgeons involved, I was like a leaf thrown about in the wind, an experiment in a test tube passed from hospital to hospital. To think now that men in white coats played God, that they sat behind closed doors and discussed the implications of mistakes in surgery, and their own improved reputations if I was a success story is disturbing. It unnerves me sixteen years later.

Teresa, an intelligent girl and a regular participant with experience in social work says, "In my view, if you analyze culture too much, you will stereotype persons with disabilities. Possibly distort their identities. Limit their successes, too." Amen.

My black, leather bag rests at my feet under the table. It is almost break time, and I plan to get a snack and a soda. I pull out some money from my wallet and hold it in my hands. On one of the flyers, I see a party will be held soon. At the bottom of the flyer, there is a black and white photo of a table with a platter of food spread before several members of the honor society. My stomach growls, a hungry feline in my body.

Before the discussion moves forward, I say, "All I know is that I don't want my minority status to determine who I am." My professor nods.

I then hear Miss Love say, "Let's take our break. Twenty minutes. Be back here."

• • •

ON OCCASION, popular bands will come to town, and if I have the money, I will rush to buy the tickets, relishing the thought of having the ridged pieces of paper between my fingers. The same tickets that excite me, though, also make me nervous at times. I guess it's the fear of losing the tickets, and the responsibility to keep an eye on them so I can take a break from the heavy workload that can be so burdensome.

I think about this when, after my psychosocial class, one of the girls says to the entire group, "We should all go to a concert sometime." The idea doesn't go over real well. I am disappointed, but, later, when I am over at the Weston Community Center picking up my mail, I notice a flyer with my favorite band on the front, the date they are coming, and the cost of the show. Inside, I am thinking, *Yes! Sweet!*

The tickets usually have a sale date, notifying me of the day I need to pick them up. I hate to admit it, but I know from experience that, if you aren't one of the first to get to the ticket office, you

GRAND MAL

don't get the good seats. Fortunately for me, the sale date this year falls on a free day, a day of no classes. So I plan to walk to the ticket office.

The Performing Arts building is all the way across campus, a long way for me to walk. I need some personal time, though. I know it. And if I don't allow myself a relaxing evening every once in a while, I might burn out. Whatever it takes is worth it.

Last year, the line was incredibly long, a slithering snake with a winding tail. It is just as long this year, if not longer, and I stand here for about two hours, moving forward as slow as a bored slug. About halfway to the ticket booth, the line comes to a halt, one of many halts, and I shuffle on my feet like John, looking at a framed board of signatures from all the famous bands that have come to town. I marvel at all the musicians' handwriting until it is my turn at the ticket booth.

• • •

NEARING THE door of my apartment, tickets in my pocket, I hear laughter. Michael's laughter. And a girl's laughter. It is surprising to hear a female voice in our pad, and my curiosity peaks. I put my hand on the knob to open the door, but it won't open. It is locked. Unusual. I consider knocking, but decide not to. Pulling out my key, and inserting it into the keyhole, I unlock the door, allowing me to enter.

I peek my head inside. "Yo!"

"Oh hey, Chris," Michael says. "How's it goin'?"

"Good." I reply. "Who's our visitor here?"

The girl is smiling broadly, hiding behind Michael. "This is Linda."

JOSHUA HOLMES

Linda is a petite girl, has long auburn hair, deep brown eyes, and a cute, crooked grin. She has stylish cat glasses balanced on a cute little nose, and a subtle hint of red lipstick on her lips. *Michael has good taste*, I think. "Hi," she says.

"Hi. Nice to meet you." I smile. When she turns away, I mouth to Michael, 'Dang! She's hot!'

I then turn, go into my room. Talk and laughter seeps under the crack in my door like an infectious gas. This continues for a couple of hours, and then all is still. When she leaves, I go out into the kitchen where Michael is cooking an Indian dish, the smell burning my nostrils. "That smells so bad, man," I say.

"But it tastes awesome. An interesting flavor," he counters. It gets quiet a minute, but, seconds later, Michael breaks the silence. "By the way, Linda told me to tell you again it was nice meeting you."

"Okay," I say. "Well thanks, I guess." I walk over to the table, and push all the chairs in. "Hey. I'm curious. Where did you meet her?"

"Met her at a restaurant. I complimented on her hair, some of her jewelry. The next thing I know, she is on break, we are talking. She tells me she is a philosophy major. I tell her I love that area of study, and we talk forever about it. We've been hanging out since." He rubs his goatee, scratches his thick unibrow. "I think we are going to go to the Dave Matthews Band concert."

"Me too. I just got back from the ticket office. Maybe you can give me a lift."

ELECTRIC

"I don't know, man. You don't think you'll have a seizure do you?" he asks. "I don't want Linda to see you have one. It might scare her away."

"You know as well as I do that I don't know when they are gonna happen. What if I do have one?" I question. "Will you avoid me to spare your girlfriend?"

He is silent, and his lack of a response makes me question our friendship.

• • •

THAT QUESTION and lack of a response upsets me. And to ease my angry feelings, I leave Michael be for a little while. During this time, though, I repeatedly tell myself I am being unreasonable, and I eventually ask him if he will accompany me to a couple places. I want him to hang with me at the Kern Graduate Building for a time, and then go down town to the gym where the karate classes are being offered. He agrees to come with me.

We opt to walk over to campus, so we are presently approaching the large walkway, a bridge above the main thoroughfare if you will, that allows us to pass over North Atherton Street. As we cross the bridge, we look at the classrooms behind glass on either side. There is a deli on the left side with a large area for everyone to sit. The Dell computer store and an art exhibit are a few steps away. On the right side, there is another lounge, and just beyond it are a Xerox copy store and the Apple computer store. It is an amazing construct. We reach the end of the bridge a minute later. We are both winded.

"Tired?" I ask Michael.

JOSHUA HOLMES

He heaves. And then he fibs. "Not a chance!"

• • •

FROM THERE we walk up Burrowes Road, a shady street lined with colonial-style fraternity and sorority houses, pass a CATA bus, the White Loop, and Waring Commons. The Kern building is around the corner from the Commons and catty corner to the Recreation Building. Inside Kern, it is packed. The vestibule opens up into a large space where several round and square tables are separated by only a foot or so. Students and faculty rush to grab the empty tables nearest to them. Long flags with the logos of all the teams we play in the Big Ten conference hang from the ceiling, and I count them, focusing on the represented teams we still haven't played this season.

Michael tugs at my arm. "There's a free table over there! Hurry or we'll lose it!"

I say, "Awesome. Perfect timing." We jog over to a table high off the ground with a set of high stools, and place our bags and coats there to save our spot.

Once he has grabbed a bagel and a caramel latte, and I have grabbed a donut and Chai tea, we awkwardly settle on our stools. I am about to apologize for getting annoyed, when he silences me. "Don't worry about it," he says. "I was the ass."

"I was just being immature." There is a curved, Indian-like pattern on the table, and I stare at it, moving my finger in a circular motion over the glazed outline.

GRAND MAL

Michael says, "It's just that she's talking to me about heavy stuff. Like long term stuff for us. Her future with me." He looks around us, trying to keep his voice low.

"Already?" I say, looking up from the table, stopping my finger motions. "I just heard you were talking to her."

"We've been talking a long time. I just decided not to tell you. Sorry." He waves his hand in the air to emphasize what he is saying. In doing so, I see a small cross tattoo under his wrist that has a red banner with the word LOVE over it. He must have had it done recently, within the past month. I think, *Man oh man, will his parents tell him he's going to hell!* But I don't say anything, for the tattoo convinces me my friend is telling the truth.

To some extent, I appreciate his honesty, so I reply, "No. It's all right. I understand."

• • •

I DO UNDERSTAND. I probably would do the same if my friend would be upset by the news. So I don't make an issue of it again. *Enough of this serious talk*, I think. *Let's have fun!* Judging from the perplexed yet hopeful expression on his face, I sense Michael agrees with me. We talk about some lighter topics while finishing up our sweets, and then leave the Kern building.

Almost forty-five minutes later, we enter the side door to the gym offering karate lessons. Our earlier talk no longer an issue. We find the office immediately. It is small, but acceptable, considering the gym isn't all that large either. On the main wall, two swords are mounted on either side of a glass encasement. The encasement glistens, protecting several large trophies. Behind a nicked table, a muscular guy with a long braided ponytail reclines in a leather chair, manning a nearby phone, and, I assume, working on finances. He asks how he can help us.

I smile and put out my hand for a shake. "I am interested in the martial arts class you are offering." He shakes my hand, almost breaks it actually (unlike Alex's shake, let me tell you!), pulls out a pamphlet, and points out with his free hand the good deals.

"Most likely I'll do the group class, but I'd like to take the free lesson first."

"Good. Good. Wise choice," he says in an authoritative, Mr. Miyagi way. Looking down at my throbbing open hand, he places the pamphlet in my palm, and then pulls at his ponytail, wrapping it up into a bun. "And what about your friend here?"

I turn to Michael. "A free lesson man. You can't beat it."

"Yeah. I guess you're right." We both make arrangements and head out with another thing to look forward to.

• • •

IN MID-JULY, the State College Arts Fest brings a lot of people to the Happy Valley. I have not experienced all the events and spectacles that make this annual festival so notorious. So, I am walking down College Avenue, passing several old houses hidden by shadows, observing students on the porches lounge, drink, and smoke. Typical activities at a party school.

About twenty houses later, I reach a mid-section where North Atherton Street and College Avenue intersect. I cross it, walk

ELECTRIC

straight ahead into the thick of things, the restaurants and shops. Normally, the students parade into stores like Abercrombie & Fitch, Eddie Bauer, McClannahan's, and Webster's bookstore. During Arts Fest week, though, with all the tents placed everywhere, and a wide array of artistic merchandise available, pottery, paintings, and jewelry, the students migrate instead to these attractions.

When I reach Allen Street, I pass the Grille, an old restaurant with decent food, looking for a nearby bench. The street is blocked off, and a stage has been erected in the middle of the road. Several people are already sitting on benches, tapping their feet as one of the local, bluegrass cover bands plays an interesting version of an Elvis hit. I enjoy the concert, sitting in a good spot that permits me to see the entire concert unobstructed. It is something different.

I am hot, real sweaty, but I want to see everything down town. When the concert ends, I decide to walk around a little more. I see students on the roofs of their Allen Street apartments observing the masses as they maneuver their way along the sidewalks. I hear children squealing, and I smell chlorinated water. I am curious, and before long, I see a platform with moving buckets of water overhead. The children don't know which bucket will tip first, so they run as fast as they can in circles to avoid the liquid content in the rotating containers. I smile to myself, enjoying the carefree atmosphere.

I near a mist machine, walk through it to cool off, and observe several food stands, lemonade stands, and smoothie stands, a sweet lover's paradise. A jazz record plays over the speakers, sounding until the next musician is ready to perform. I get a milkshake at a nearby ice cream shop, and decide to head home. I am glad I went, and will return to the Arts Fest later this weekend.

• • •

ONLY UNTIL I walk out of the elevator just outside my apartment door do I forget Michael's debate team will be having a group session. Why they chose to do this over hanging with the masses at Arts Fest is beyond me, but I guess each person places value on something different. *What a shame*, I think.

If I remember correctly, the topic at hand is Plato and the allegory of the man who twice enters the cave with all the slaves.

I decide I'll sit with them. I have nothing else to do, and I might as well observe why Michael hosts this particular activity. You know, I have already stated why I believe he joined this group. His family life. To spite his parents. What I am still not convinced about is whether he enjoys questioning truth. He says so, but I find it hard to believe someone who once lived by absolutes, no matter how stringent, can, later in life, fully be content as a relativist.

By now, Michael, John, and Alex have moved our kitchen table out into the hall, and have set up the couches so they can face one another. The couches are bland and hard, a dull shade of grey with pillows that feel like wood. But it'll have to do. And the table! It is bent. A tree would be embarrassed! Nevertheless, they are all settled and ready to begin.

"So," Linda says, her cat glasses at the tip of her nose. "Where did we leave off?"

GRAND MAL

Michael says, "At the most interesting part! The cave and the shadows." His one thick eyebrow goes up like a puppy's ear when waiting on a treat. He then feels the highlighter behind his ear, his father's regimented training so obvious.

Linda eloquently says, "Yes. When these chained people are in the dark and can only see their shadows. For them, it is the only reality that exists."

"Hmmmm. Yet there are more than the shadows." Alex retorts antagonistically, wagging his pudgy finger in the air, his forehead extremely creased. "There is a wall, a fire, and wanderers with jars in hand. They don't help them, but they are also in the cave. Ha! So, there you go! Another reality!"

"So, what is real?" asks John, a bit edgy in his seat. "What is the truth?"

"That is the question John. That is why we are here!" says Michael, who I notice is making sure his watch covers the tattoo.

And so they all begin pondering these questions. They banter some, and I hear Alex say, "True" several more times. I get aggravated not only by his mantra, but also at the pointless nature of debating. What purpose does it serve?

I wonder about this for a reason. From experience, I know the die-hard analyst, whether it is a member of the press or an educated average Joe, likes to take a truth, and tear it apart so there is no reliable explanation for the subject in question. And what is interesting to me, and I have seen it repeatedly, on TV and here at school, is the fact that, in the end, some of the analysts don't really know what they believe, if in fact they ever did. And that, in my opinion, is reality.

JOSHUA HOLMES

When the debaters are done talking about the allegory, they relate the same principles to their own lives.

Alex says, "My definition of a good Parent is obviously different than my own Parents' definition. And my idea of verbal abuse is different than the ideas of my Grandparents."

"Along the same lines, Alex," John replies, shaking his head in agreement. "My Parents and I believe my peers at school abused me to get back at my Mother, but my bullies might have been doing it because they were cruel by nature. Who knows?"

Linda says, "Well. Plato's allegory gives us plenty to think about. That's for sure."

I agree. And from what I gather, the man in the allegory comes out of the cave more confused about reality than when he went inside, the sun beating down on him as he tries to reach enlightenment and find the truth.

• • •

THE SUN beats down on me, the light reflecting off my glasses like a mirror shimmering against a vase. I squint, cup my hands around my eyes to see through the strobes, and head for the shadows to ward off the heat. The air is still, no breeze at all, the Happy Valley as arid as a desert. It has been dry for a while, and a change in the weather is inevitable. I see cumulus clouds in the distance. *It's going to storm*, I think. *It's just a matter of time.*

On Allen Street again, I see the storeowners and employees are taking advantage of all the tourists visiting State College for the Arts Fest. They have set up outdoor clothing racks and boxes full of

ELECTRIC

over-stocked hats, shorts, shirts, sweatshirts, sweatpants, and even jackets. Prices range from five dollars to seventy-five dollars. Not bad, I guess. As I look through the selection, though, I can't help but wonder whether the retailers jacked up the initial costs to make all of these items look like a steal. I guess they would be stupid not to.

So I won't spend money carelessly, I walk towards campus to see the talented artists from around the country manning more tents. Artists who sell some products at unimaginable prices. There are so many items and trinkets here at Arts Fest it could take multiple visits to see everything. I do manage to see a lot, however.

• • •

ONCE I'VE finished looking around the remaining tents on campus, I am inspired to draw. I have seen abstract lithographs, beautiful photography, impressionistic landscape paintings, and realistic portrait drawings. While I am eager to get my creative juices flowing, I wait, and return to Webster's bookstore. I spend hours here, no matter the time, weather, or season.

I have my own favorite section of the bookstore, a remote area towards the back in a cubicle-shaped box of bookshelves. I sit on a small bench, and swivel my body around to survey the used, but average, selection of novels. I soak up the smell of the novels, the pungent, sour odor of mildewed paper. A nasty smell to some, but a familiar and appreciated scent for me.

I also smell hot chocolate, cappuccino, and fruit. The smell is coming from the front of the building. "Mmmmmmmm," I mutter to myself. *Man, I could go for a smoothie*. I haven't yet had one today, so I decide to get the treat. Besides, I have to go up front anyway, to talk to Sam, a mentor of mine.

On my way to the front of the store, I look at a variety of average pictures on the walls by some local artist I've never heard of. A different series of pictures is placed on the same walls weekly, and I wonder whether Sam would allow me to showcase my own artwork at some point. Not to be cocky, but I think I am a lot better than this guy.

Anyway, in the front of the store, Sam stands behind a coffee bar, a small café. He has thick glasses, a goatee, and long dreads that drape over his tie-dye shirt. He is sort of eccentric, loud, and loose with his tongue. I sometimes think he spikes his coffee and overdrinks, but he has always been nice to me, a good conversationalist who offers good advice.

I usually come here to write my master's paper on my laptop, to escape the miserable weather and relax, but, today, I have come to hear Sam's take on Michael's comment about my seizing in front of his girlfriend. I swivel in my little corner for about an hour, but I eventually walk to the front of the store and find a table to sit at, only a short distance away from the coffee bar.

No one is giving Sam business today, so I purchase the smoothie, a strawberry ice cream drink. Sam brings the smoothie over to me in his bare feet, limping. He was injured in Vietnam, was shot in the knee. His shoulders sag, his weariness obvious. He says, "What's happenin' young chap?"

"Nothing much. Just enjoying the Arts Fest."

GRAND MAL

"I bought a new bike, ya know." I shake my head in awe. This man is something. He has a big Cadillac at home, but he chooses to cycle to work everyday. In sandals! "I customized it," he goes on. "Looks like a Harley now." He chuckles as he pulls a chair out to sit with me. He props his leg up on a nearby table.

A rich man, Sam sees no reason to make a show of it. He inherited his riches, and he could easily act aloof, as if he is above us all. But he isn't. His humility is refreshing to those who know him. It is refreshing to me. Yet because he doesn't display his worth, he lost his wife, who evidently married him for his money.

To make his life even emptier, his wife took Sam's kid away. She filed for custody, after he returned from war, and won. He never saw him again, despite his efforts to get visitation. All Sam has left are memories from when his son was young. He has repeatedly told me he wished he had adopted after the divorce.

"A Harley?" I say. "Good for you. Your other bike was looking pretty pitiful." He emphatically nods. Looking down, I glance at his deformed leg, but turn away so I don't appear to be staring. I add, "Now all you need are some shoes."

"No way, lad. Shoes are for sissies." I look at his leg again. Sam once told me his wife had changed when he came home "a cripple". He believes she expected him to die and resented she couldn't live as a wealthy widow. This makes me sad for him.

"Tell me, Sam," I say. "Has anyone ever insinuated he or she wouldn't hang with you because of your injury?"

"One of the guys I shot in Vietnam!" He guffaws.

"No. Seriously."

"I guess. My ex-wife actually," he says. "I never really acknowledge rude people, though."

"My best friend is falling for a girl, and I think he wants me to stay away because of my seizures." I think, *Well he denied it, but still.*

Sam looks at an antique painting that hangs on the wall behind me. "Don't let it get you down, chap. You are too strong for that."

"But he's my best friend . . ." I take a deep breath, inhale deeply, and a waft of mildew and coffee envelopes me.

"Friends will come and go," he says. "As the saying goes, seasons change."

• • •

PART TWO:

FALL SEMESTER SEASONS CHANGE

SAM WAS right about the changing seasons, for summer has ended and fall is beckoning. The sun has stopped shining on a frequent basis and the wind calls out as rain falls, thunder rolls, and lightning cracks. The temperature is dropping. The students, myself included, no longer wear short-sleeved shirts. I have pulled out my black pea coat.

People aren't smiling as they do in the summer, the weather pretty depressing. I see many people running to their cars under umbrellas, squinting, and I am now one of those students keeping dry under the Patee-Paterno Library overhang, waiting for the CATA bus to arrive.

JOSHUA HOLMES

The green leaves on the trees have turned shades of gold, orange, and red. The leaves that have fallen from the oak canopies suffocate the earth's surface, preventing the grass to breathe, yellowing the reeds as they wither.

I hate getting out of bed some mornings.

One thing, however, that lifts my spirits is the opening of football season, watching the improved players I saw at the Blue and White game, at the pep rallies at the Recreation Building and Beaver Stadium. One day, sometime in June, when it was still summer, I also bought season tickets to watch the Nittany Lion football team play. Considering season tickets sell so quickly, I was fortunate.

When we play our most rivaled nemesis, the Ohio State Buckeyes, hordes of people, small children, adolescents, college students, parents, and grandparents, flood the sidewalks. Some of them walk down Curtin, Bigler, and Pollock Roads at a vigorous pace, in attempts to be the first to arrive at the front gates of Beaver Stadium.

There are always people scalping tickets outside the front gates, most of whom will hold the tickets up in the air waving them back and forth, calling out, "Selling tickets here!" Some will negotiate the sale price; some won't budge. It enlivens the atmosphere.

Every couple of feet, there are Penn State Bookstore stands filled with shirts, hats, cups, cheering items, and school programs. The sales representatives are running around disheveled, trying to keep up, gathering various purchases.

For me, there is no hurry, since, as the football ticket reads, I am a senior, eligible to watch the game in the student section, the S zone. Funny, thinking about it, even when I want to hurry, it is dif-

GRAND MAL

ficult, the masses a briar patch that snags me as I push forward. As soon as the gates open, and I am at the front of the line, I exchange my ticket for another with a specific row and number in which to sit, most of the time on the thirty-yard line.

I recall the day Michael made the high school football team. It was a turning point in his academic career. Now seizure free, he didn't have to worry about any outside stimuli that might have preceded a neurological reaction. The scar on his head was his trademark, he told me once. The distinct feature he was known for in the locker room.

Meanwhile, on the sidelines, I rubbed my scar and cheered him on. Michael was the starting quarterback, my favorite position. Unfortunately, I still had to worry about overheating and atmospheric stimulation that could start a seizure. These factors never kept me from attending the games. I loved it, and I love attending games today.

I did have an advantage over Michael when he was playing, though. I spoke with the beautiful Mary Grace, who had grown into an attractive young lady with a wonderful smile, and a quiet, almost meek, demeanor. She was even more attractive than when she was in middle school; having a slender curvaceous figure, light smooth skin, and a full face with high cheekbones. Better yet, her personality impressed me.

Mary Grace had no interest in popularity, refrained from complaining, and didn't compare herself to others to justify her actions. She had plans to be a nurse, and, she told me, nothing was going to get in her way. She was the real thing. Still is, I believe.

Anyway, she settled on the bleacher next to me, talking to me about her school day, and questioning about mine. We had a good time even when our school day was rough, and I felt proud sitting next to a pretty blonde with a great body. I never told her that, though.

Once inside the Beaver Stadium gate, I head towards a hotdog stand, a concrete booth with chip displays on the counter, and a big, blue board on the wall with all the menu items. There are several booths, each of which are somewhat hidden by the crowd, but I go to the one nearest to my seat and wait my turn.

• • •

IT IS hard to describe the magnitude of Beaver Stadium, the mere size of it. I'm pretty sure it holds 110 thousand fans. Every student here in State College who loves football, and who hasn't had the opportunity to experience the rush I get when I am in the third row of the student section, hasn't a clue of the power of Penn State spirit. There is nothing like it.

Initially, before the game starts, the most exciting thing for me is finding the seat, especially when I am right behind the players. I know I am thrilled when the staff walks up the ramp with me, and finds my place. At this point, the stadium isn't all that full. There is a faint smell of popcorn in the air, mixed with a hint of nachos and cheese. It takes a while for me to grow accustomed to the different odors.

Normally, I hand in the ticket two hours in advance, and once inside the stadium, I can't leave until the game is over. It works out perfectly, though, because I get to watch each team exercise, stretch, and practice different plays, the quarterback passing one ball to different receivers, the kicker repeatedly punting another ball across the field. The latest rap music blares, revving up the fans more and more

ELECTRIC

as the hours pass, the replays of past games on the monitors instigating cheers.

About forty-five minutes before game time, Joe Paterno jogs out in his blue windbreaker and waves to the crowd, his notorious thick glasses accentuating his classic nose. He then claps as he talks with his assistant coaches on the sidelines. They jog back under the stadium, into the locker room after they have made their appearances.

Announcements are made, sponsors are acknowledged, and on occasion, other Penn State sports teams are called onto the field, recognized for an achievement, receiving an award. It is filler, of course, but nice to see nonetheless.

I get all riled up when I see the Penn State dancers kicking their legs up in the air in unison. They are dressed in short, dark blue sweaters and even shorter skirts. I check out each girl, observe her physique, and often think, *Come to papa!*

When the Blue Band marches out on the field in unison, the drummers, trombonists, trumpeters, and saxophonists forming the letters P, S, and U on the turf as they play the Alumni song, Hail to the Lion, I marvel, imagining the hours of practice that contribute to the band's synchronization. Their march usually brings in all the people, which means it is time to stand.

I really don't know why they call the benches in the student section seats, because you really don't sit at all during the five-hour game. Just about every student is either hopping up and down to encourage the Nittany Lions, screaming to distract the opposition and chanting negative phrases to taunt, or dancing and singing to music after we score.

JOSHUA HOLMES

When I think about the kind of person I am normally, sober and reserved, and the kind of person I am in the stands, a loud, antagonistic, emotional roller coaster, sometimes quaking out of anger and nervousness, I just have to shake my head. How can sports make me act like this?

The answer is easy. Penn State spirit. When I yell 'Go Joe!' or shout 'Joepa! Joepa!' or 'We are Penn State!' with thousands of people, even the bare-chested guys with shaggy, blue and white hair and painted faces, a sense of camaraderie washes over me, a sense of belonging. It puts a lump in my throat, and brings a smile to my face, an unfamiliar joy.

• • •

WHEN THE game is over and we have won, I am so wound up I have to take a deep breath. Several, actually. There is an ambulance out front of the stadium, and the lights are flashing, red lights rapidly flickering across my face, colorful bullets firing at my retinas. I begin to feel funny, hollow in my eyes, and sick to my stomach. "Shoot!" I mutter. "Here we go again." My auras always start at the most inopportune times.

I know I have to get down, on the ground as soon as possible. But where? Thousands of aggressive people are brushing against me, trying to pass me. There's no place for my preservation. Unless I can reach the group of parked campers, where all the tailgaters are. There are patches of grass there too. I walk with the crowd, still hoping I can make it.

GRAND MAL

Soon I see some grass, some tailgaters, but I know the electricity in my head is spreading, and I won't be able to hold out much longer. I see a few lounge chairs sitting ahead of me. Close by, two men with bloated guts are drinking beer, laughing loudly, and a boy is throwing a football in the air, and running to catch his own pass. I lay myself on the ground, right next to a camper. Someone is bound to find me.

Just as there was a time in my life when I dreamed or imagined certain situations in the color blue, I also had nightmares in shades of red. It only took minimal exposure to any color of red during my seizures to bring about a horrible, but plausible, nightmare. In my nightmares of red, I am falling eternally, only from the sky this time. I can't stop myself, gravity's mighty pull once again at work.

I have access to a red parachute, but it won't open, surges of fear pummeling my entire body. I search the backpack that tugs on my shoulders, looking for the cord that will trigger the parachute to unfold, to no avail.

A man in a red jumpsuit above me, also falling, yells at me, saying I am not listening. "You are doing it wrong, Chris. What's the matter with you?" I keep trying, but I miss the cord, the extension too limp.

The man has a devilish quality about him, glassy eyes, a contorted mouth with visible fangs, and fingers like talons. He aggressively claws the air, trying to grab my bag so I don't continue to drop, rapidly falling towards the earth. His hellish body is out of control, and the parachute he is floating under is starting to deflate, putting him in more danger than myself.

JOSHUA HOLMES

I see flocks of vultures soaring around us, avoiding us almost, but ready to feast on us if we perish. I also see exhaust lines from a plane in the distance. Why can't they help us?

I fall and fall and fall, the red clay earth approaching at an ever-increasing speed.

Next to the camper, my right arm is shaking hard, slamming against the aluminum siding. My mouth is touching the earth, red sod on my tongue. I grunt as I try to breathe, but all I get are brief whiffs of rubber from the rear tire. Spittle lines my lips. I feel a hand with long fingernails on my shoulder a moment later, and I hear myself yell out. One of the men with bloated guts hovers over me, the boy throwing the ball asking, "What's wrong with him?"

• • •

I AM A dead weight. A barbell. There is confusion all around me. The man is not a lifter, and has trouble maneuvering around me, unsure how to help me. I wonder why I am always found by the uninformed.

I feel as if I have been pelted by pieces of hail, my muscles bruised and strained by falls and solid crystals of weakness. The man says, "Take it easy, son. I'm here to help." The nerve of the guy! Telling me to take it easy. *Trade places with me for a few hours, and then shoot your mouth, buddy*, I think. *Can't you see me, here? I can't do a darn thing!*

I am now on my back, the worst position to be in when having a Grand Mal. For a moment, I had a surge of energy, and I got in a sitting position. I leaned on my wrists, which were trembling under

ELECTRIC

the pressure, and I tried to lean forward. But my wrists buckled, and I fell sideways. Another surge of energy, and another failed attempt. I fell backwards, thus my current position.

I feel as if I am suffocating. I see bodies surrounding me, hear shuffling feet that sound like combat boots in action, constant motion. And I can't move. I get panicked. Incredibly panicked. I begin to whimper out of fear, my lips quivering. My body goes rigid, and I look from face to face, helpless and breathless.

• • •

IRONICALLY, THE same ambulance that started my seizure has come to save me; that's what the EMTs think, anyway. The vehicle is only a few feet away from me, and I dread what the people inside will soon do to me.

I want them to leave me be. Let me recover on my own. I don't want them to interfere. All my adult life, I have had to accept, if I am found by EMTs, they will want to involve medical staff at the nearest hospitals. I have had to accept they might have me lie down on a wooden pallet, and the possibility they might tie me down, wrapping me in buckles, even though I want to go home.

The lights are still flashing, and I have to wait. The wait is horrible.

• • •

I AM FORTUNATE. The EMTs don't buckle me down. I am wet and weak, though; my head is in pain, exploding like an active volcano. My body takes about forty-five minutes to rebound, and when I am fully functioning, I just want to get out of there. I sign the release forms, and begin towards Webster's bookstore. I have to lean on someone. Michael won't want to help, I don't think. He might be embarrassed.

It takes me longer to get there. I am still wobbly, and I am still breathing heavily. No big surprise. My rib cage was contracted for almost an hour. When I walk in, I see Sam wiping down the tables. I collapse onto a nearby chair.

The bookstore has grown, and I am happy about this. It means people are purchasing a lot of text. A number of new shelves full of books have been erected, and the lounging area has been rearranged. Sitting here, I think, *Chris! You are nuts! Go home!* But I have no one to go home to. I need someone to show me some sympathy. The exact same thing I normally don't want people to give me. Very contradictory, don't you think?

Sam doesn't turn around. He continues to scrub, his dreads falling around his face with every push of the dust rag. "We're gonna be closing soon, champ," he says, not realizing it is me.

"That a new tie dye shirt, Sam?" I say, still a bit breathless. "Very colorful."

He turns, looks at me more closely. "Chris, my friend. Sorry. I didn't know it was you." I tell him it's all right.

"You look like trash," he impulsively says. "What's up?"

"Just had a seizure. And I feel like trash."

"So, chap, why are you not home sleeping?"

"I thought about it, but I figured you would make me a free smoothie and lift my spirits."

GRAND MAL

He puts the rag in his pocket and walks behind the counter, pulls out his blender and scoops some ice cream. He then picks out a couple bananas and strawberries and mixes it with the ice cream. The blender roars as it softens the mixture. "When my boy was little. He was as stubborn as you are today. And if I didn't know better," he practically yells. "I'd think you were a mooch."

"Thanks," I say sarcastically, shaking my head. "I feel so much better."

"So. Tell me, was this seizure stress related?"

"I don't think so. The ambulance lights at the game did it, I think."

"I was just curious." He puts whip cream on my smoothie, and walks over to me. I grab the cup. "Considering how upset you've been with Michael."

I close my eyes, and put my head in my hands. "Yeah. He's been bothering me. But I don't think this seizure had anything to do with it."

• • •

I AM BEAT this morning from the seizure at the game, and I almost stay in bed, but I get up. I make a decision I won't let my seizure hold me back. This is a decision I face daily. I feel horrible, but I arrive to the Chambers building for class on time. And I soak up some of the information given me.

My head is still aching; when I cough, laugh, or bend over, I cringe, an avalanche of pain plummeting over the dips in my skull. I deal with it, though. There are about twenty people surrounding me, all of them in individual seats wrapped around the room in a circle. There are people of different cultural backgrounds: Indian,

JOSHUA HOLMES

African American, and Caucasian mostly. Some Asian and African. The multicultural class consists of people in different programs outside my own. There are computers scattered against the walls, a table in the center of the room, and a chalkboard lined with children's crafts. I sit in the back, closest to the door, incredibly anxious to leave.

The whole class revs me up inside. I have a bad attitude. I am sick of it. The professors are intent on showing me how unfair life is for minorities. I get it. I understand people have feelings, have troubles as a result of others' behaviors, but I just can't believe the curriculum, the repeated emphasis on the fact that certain groups of people can't make it, that special treatment is necessary otherwise it is discrimination. Discrimination, my ass! I know discrimination exists, but using it as a crutch is not productive. How am I, as a counselor, supposed to empower clients, the whole point of counseling, if all I hear is clients will only be a success if they aren't discriminated against and are privileged?

I think every person is capable to be the best. Color, gender, and disability, in my case, may be setbacks, big setbacks, and they will make life hard, but, with help, I believe anyone can be a success. Instead, here I am, listening to some professors complain about their place in society, stereotyping people while preaching to do the opposite, playing the blame game.

I speak up. "It just seems like the minority in here are more hostile than the majority group, and the majority group . . ." I make quotation marks with my fingers. "Have been ripped apart for the past three hours." Someone objects to my comment, and I con-

ELECTRIC

tinue. "It would be one thing if we were talking about discrimination in the thirties, here."

I may be overly-sensitive because I am a minority, and I have succeeded despite my privilege, or lack thereof. I like the thought of having control over my life, and it eats me up when I hear people say otherwise. It also eats me up, because I know life is hard, and I don't need an educational institution to remind me of that. My daily life as a person with Epilepsy is reminder enough. Pain as a result of my seizures is reminder enough. Fear as a result of my seizures is reminder enough. Unwanted attention as a result of my seizures is reminder enough. Social and transportation setbacks as a result of my seizures are reminder enough. I know people with Epilepsy face difficulties, but no one hears us complaining, asking for special treatment.

When this class ends, I know my head will hurt worse than when I arrived. Three stinking hours of pessimism and promotion of division, generalizations and heated debate. But it has been good in one respect. The class has validated my self-confidence, and my confidence in others with Epilepsy.

• • •

TO ALLEVIATE my annoyance, I head to the gym where I took my first lesson, where I am now learning Kali, the Filipino martial arts. I am finally participating in a sport of sorts. Now that I am involved in a physical activity, I think there is no better way to rid of my negative emotions than to use it to advance my proficiency.

JOSHUA HOLMES

The gym is in behind a pizza shop. It is a fairly large, open space with a boxing ring in the center, and a loft covered in wrestling mats where I have class Tuesdays and Thursdays. I take the class with about seven other students. I have been taking it a while, but I have a lot of room for improvement.

Michael had been taking the class with me. We always walked home together, congratulating each other on a win during our competitions, or empathizing with one another if either of us lost.

That was before Linda came along and stopped it. One day towards the end of the summer, three months after Linda and Michael met, Michael said to me, "Linda is afraid I will hurt myself. She wants me to stop fighting."

He explained that Linda appreciated intellect over physical brawn, that her mom raised her as an only child that way, and she'd been taught to resolve problems through discussion versus through any physical means.

You see, Michael informed me Linda hasn't always been attractive. At one point, she had numerous blemishes, and was pretty thick in the mid-section. She often came home crying because boys made fun of her, had hit her, or thrown rocks at her. At first, she responded in the same fashion, but it only made things worse. Only when she saw her mother address and successfully settle the situation with the other parents, did she realize it was better to be diplomatic about troubling circumstances. Thus, in her opinion, Michael told me, Linda felt he'd be more prone to act out physically if he continued training in the martial arts; especially Kali, since it is probably the most violent form out there.

GRAND MAL

"Well, what are you going to do?" I asked. "You love this, man. And it's not like you're training to beat up people who disagree with you!"

"I know, Chris, I know," he said. "But I think Linda might be the one. And I don't want to lose her."

"You do what you gotta do, man."

"Every time I went to karate class with you, she worried," Michael said. "She would rub my scar afterwards and say she didn't want me to have another one." *He used to love it in high school when the jocks complimented him on his scar*, I thought. *It's amazing what a girl will do to you.*

"Just think about it before you quit, " I said. "You've worked hard to get where you are." He had already made up his mind, though. He just wanted to hear what I had to say.

I think about this as I stretch my body, loosening my limbs to lift weights. I walk over to the weight room and get some twenty-pounders. Metal hits metal as a lifter places a heavy weight in its cradle. I sit down on a nearby bench and do some curls, determined to work through the burn. It is so easy to give in for me, but I have fortitude. I have always been a determined person, and I don't plan on changing in this respect.

I hear the bell ring in the background, sounding the end of a boxing match for a couple of men working out. The bell sounds frequently, and at times gets irritating when jumping around, sweating profusely, trying to concentrate in the sweltering heat.

I curl for a half hour, and move onto my karate moves. By the time I have finished practicing with my sparring sticks, and I have repeated my footwork matrix numerous times, my mind is clear. I feel revived and excited about my progress. Sort of proud, too. I can now go home and rest without resentful thoughts.

• • •

MOMENTS AFTER I have walked into my apartment and collapsed on the chair in my room, I hear what sounds like a herd of stampeding elephants, but what I have come to know as several people running up the stairwell to the third floor. Moments after that, I hear the herd snorting outside my door. And then in my living room. I forgot again that it is debate night.

I hear Linda say, "Okay. Tonight it's Aristotle." *Another discussion about reality*, I think to myself. *Thank God I did some research.*

"Yeah. Potentiality vs. actuality." Alex says. "I don't know if I buy it. And I bet you, Michael, that you can't win me over." More pessimism.

Michael looks at Alex, his brow furrowed. "The existence of anything has to have a cause, right?"

"According to Aristotle anyway!" John adds, punching his left fist into his right hand over and over again, as jittery as ever.

Ever the pacifist diplomat, Linda takes a sip of drink from one of my cups, root beer I think, then intervenes, "Now, now, boys. No need to be harsh." Her mom would be proud.

"Well, Michael starts. "There are four causes. The material cause. The efficient cause. The formal cause. And the final cause."

"True. True." Alex says, his forehead creased. "I'll give you that much." He continues, "But as far as I'm concerned, I'm not the

ELECTRIC

cause of a life without a true family. It's not my fault my parents never were, and my grandparents are jerks!"

"And my mother caused me to run away from bullies. Not me," John adds. Everything is quiet. I'm telling you, it is an intense moment; time for my entrance. "Hey Chris!!" they all exclaim when they see me.

"Yo! You want to hear my thoughts?"

"Sure," they say in unison.

"Before I begin, I'd like to preface that you are looking at the concepts circumstantially, whereas I am looking at them materially." They all nod, encouraging me to keep talking.

"When I graduate," I announce, walking into the room. "My diploma will prove actuality." I go to the cupboard, get a cup of my own, and pour some root beer to quench my thirst.

"How so?" John wonders.

"It will exist on bond paper, proof of material cause. It will have been previously printed on the paper, proof of efficient cause. The Deans and President will have signed it and a stamp of completion will symbolize what it is, proof of formal cause. And it is the last formal document I'll receive from the university, proof of final cause."

"Impressive!" Linda squeals. "Very Impressive. Don't you think guys?"

"A very interesting analogy," Michael says, nodding.

John stops punching his hand. He seems at peace with what I've said. He wipes some sweat from his shiny forehead and smiles a little, grabs a Frito from a recently opened bag.

Alex rolls his eyes, but concedes, "Okay. You have a point."

• • •

JOSHUA HOLMES

TONIGHT, THE same pillow that cradles my head turns into an adhesive. I wake up, and my head is a brick cemented by cotton mortar. I try to lift my head, but it doesn't move. Again, I am powerless. Depending on the night, the pillow won't let go for long periods of time. Other nights, I might only be stuck momentarily. Either way it is an awful experience.

I try to prop myself up, but I am unable. It is even worse when my mouth is inhaling the pillowcase. I try to spit the cloth from my mouth, and I get saliva everywhere. So, not only am I inhaling a pillowcase, I am inhaling a wet pillowcase. I sweat heavily, and I hear myself pant.

I am not exactly sure why my head won't move, but it only makes sense I have had a seizure that I was unaware of, and I am in my Postictal period, my motor skills in recovery. When I have the seizures at night, my nightmares are the most vivid, and probably more repetitive than a back-to-back, horror movie marathon.

I repeatedly dream about tornadoes, and how helpless I am. I run around looking for cover. I see through a window three dark funnel clouds ripping up the earth, houses split down the middle like tree trunks sawed in half. The window frame starts to shake, the wood beginning to peel, the paint chipping.

I can feel the force, even though the eye hasn't touched. I run around my apartment, look for a safe place in a closet under a stairwell. It is full. I run to my bed, to see if I can fit underneath. It is too low to the ground. I hear a voice yell, "Not there, Chris. You are gonna kill yourself! Over here!" At the same time, I hear another voice say, "There's no time to listen to him! Do what needs to be

GRAND MAL

done!" But I don't know what needs to be done. So I run throughout the apartment, looking under the kitchen table, and then the cabinets under the sink. I even consider just lying on the ground, my stomach and face against the floor, in the same position I am in as I wait for my head to detach from my pillow.

Things start to fall, the ceiling fan, my lamps, the pictures I have spent hours drawing. And then it happens. The window frame gives in. The glass is thrust forward by the pressure, shattering everywhere. Shards surround me. Somehow I am still alive, and I look up through what used to be a window, just an opening now making me even more vulnerable.

I see debris thrown about. I see people and animals sucked up, killed, and spit out as though Mother Nature doesn't like the taste of them. I live through my dreams, but what makes them so horrible is that the twisters hover. They don't subside, and one wrong move on my part could seal my demise.

Only when a lot of the cotton mortar disintegrates can I lift my head up off the pillow, and I can sit up. I am fed up, and I ask God why this won't end. No reply.

• • •

WHEN I don't hear a reply, it angers me. I punch my pillow. I sit there in the dark, and ask myself out loud why I can't be normal. Why can't I live a day without a darn physical problem? Sleep through a night without excess brain activity? It just sucks so badly sometimes, I become hopeless. It isn't fair! Why do I have to exist like this?

JOSHUA HOLMES

At the same time, though it is hard to believe, I say, "Chris! Cut it out! Snap out of it!" I try to convince myself things could be worse. I've made it this far. I have lived through more pain and confusion than many have.

I think I am not dealt more than I can handle. I will make it. Tomorrow is a new day. Probably another day of auras. My seizures might get worse, but things are bound to improve. I have no clue what is the explanation for my condition, but I have Epilepsy for a reason. This statement is all I have to fall back on.

Hunched over, I sigh and shake my head. For whatever reason, I haven't gotten a sensible response from above for sixteen years. Figures.

• • •

DOESN'T LIFE just work like this, though? *Just when I am about to lose it*, I think, rolling my eyes, *something happens*. After sixteen years of trying to mix, match, and balance medicines, my neurologist calls me early this morning, just as I am drifting off, to tell me a new drug is out that, in his opinion, will control my seizures. Should I believe it and take it at face value, or brush the possibility aside? I've been let down by the medical community so often, I am apprehensive to trust anything doctors and nurses say. Believe me, I want to trust them. I do.

"So Chris. Are you still there?"

"Yeah. I'm here."

"Sorry to call so early, Chris. But I think there is a possibility we could take care of your seizures."

ELECTRIC

"No. It's all right. I'm up," I say, cradling the phone in the crux of my neck as I lean against the wall. "I had a rough night, a bad seizure, so this is good news."

"Well, as soon as you can get home, make an appointment, and come to the office."

"I'll do that." Maybe. I then turn the phone off and lay it on the ground, curl up under the covers, and fall asleep.

• • •

PART THREE:

YEAR TWO, SPRING SEMESTER, SEASONS END

I USUALLY ONLY get in a few hours of sleep after I recover my motor skills. I am exhausted, but I fear getting stuck again. So, once more, I don't get enough rest. Oh well. *I'll be dragging today*, I think. And early calls don't help enliven me any.

As I open my bedroom door on a Saturday morning following one of these episodes, I rub my eyes. I soon see Michael in the kitchen dressed only in boxers, making wonderful smelling pancakes. He has out syrup and butter, and my stomach mutters a desperate utterance.

JOSHUA HOLMES

"Hey Michael," I say, still rubbing the sleep out of my eyes. He has a grin on his face, an expression I usually see when he is thinking about his girlfriend.

"Hi."

I see a reflection from an unknown source on the wall, and I look around until I realize it is coming from Michael. He has a new earring. It is a gold stud, nothing special in my opinion, but a significant change for Michael. What an evil boy. I refrain from commenting on his change in style. I know he wants me to, but I decide not to talk about it, for it is his ear. Not mine. Besides that, I see someone else is here.

Linda walks out of Michael's room in a nighty. "Good morning, Chris." I try to flatten my hair, to make myself presentable. It is all over the place. I am shocked she is here at the apartment so early, but I don't show it. Had they slept with each other already? *I shouldn't really be surprised*, I think. *These days, it is so commonplace.*

"Morning," I reply.

Michael says to me, "Linda and I are going to visit her parents today." He places a stack of pancakes on a plate. "I haven't met them yet, Chris." I nod in acknowledgement. I think, *Wow, things are getting very serious between them now!* It sucks he is paying me less attention all the time. But, hey, that is his prerogative.

"Well," I say without sincerity. "I hope you have a good time."

"It should be interesting."

Michael and I usually went to a matinee on Saturdays, but that changed when Linda arrived, too. They go together now. I go by myself. Don't get me wrong, I enjoy my personal time; it is just hard

ELECTRIC

letting go of traditions. I am a regimented person, routine-oriented, and any kind of change throws me off. Linda has brought so much change. I am having difficulty adjusting to college life without my best friend.

They sit down to eat with each other, converse as if I'm not in the room. She tells Michael about her parents. Uninterested, I go into the bathroom to take my medication and shower. I know it might sound funny, but I am feeling more and more alienated.

• • •

WHEN I feel neglected, I tend to retreat and draw. It is hard to explain, but I get this innate feeling that motivates me to create something, and, if I don't express myself, I get uncomfortable. Feelings of neglect and discomfort are counterproductive, so I decide to head out to Old Main again.

I was in a groove this past summer, but with a new set of classes scheduled, I was forced to reprioritize, to shift my focus back to my academic responsibilities. Everyone has to take a breather, though. At least I do. So, with that said, I collect my art supplies and head out, leaving Michael and Linda to their discussion over pancakes.

Over the past couple months I have collected a few photos I would like to duplicate in pastel, with my own personal twist, to be sure. I like drawing the elderly. I find it challenging to perfect wrinkles and folds in the skin, long intricate beards, and straw hats. So, I have some drawing options today.

JOSHUA HOLMES

On the way to Old Main, I observe a group of high school kids and their parents watch a tour guide as he walks backwards pointing to significant locales, and listen to him speak of the benefits associated with the university. They all shout, "We are . . . Penn State!!" The hopeful expressions on their faces remind me of how excited I was when I first took the tour with Michael.

Ignoring the tour guide, Michael said to me then, "We get through this school, man, and we are set."

I thoughtfully said, "Yeah. But it won't be easy."

"We want it bad, though," he said softly.

"You've got that right."

That conversation sticks out to me, because I can recall how academically driven Michael was. I haven't heard him talk of classes since he met Linda. But, you know, who am I to question his motivation?

Anyway, it is a fifteen-minute walk from White Course to Old Main, and it takes a lot of my energy to make it to my bench under the oaks without dropping my supplies. I only observe the group taking the tour briefly, and then I continue to my destination. I don't really know what my creativity will lead to this afternoon, but I'm sure it will amount to something. I won't be drawing a girl who reminds me of Mary Grace, but a stimulating person nonetheless.

• • •

ON MY way home, that foul taste in my mouth, the second kind of aura I experience, manifests itself behind my left molars. It really is bizarre, the sensations I sometimes get when I am in the early stage of a seizure. My mouth feels pasty, almost like peanut butter,

GRAND MAL

and wet with bubbles. For some reason I grind my teeth and stare for a period.

I then stop in mid-stride, still grinding and staring. For a moment, I come to, and I try to speak. "Chri . . .ss." I slowly and intently say, consciously trying to overcome the looming seizure. "You . . . Uh." I lose my ability to speak. There is a glitch in the system upstairs. Then, alright again, I try once more, "Chri . . . ss. You. Can. Maaaa . . Uh . . . Make it." The sensation then leaves me. My mouth doesn't feel sticky anymore, and my molars are free of bubbles. I say out loud, "Thank you God."

Okay. I am back to myself for the time being. I look straight ahead, but I try not to stare at anything. Too much staring is sure to start up this episode again. I look at everything skittishly, the sidewalk for a minute, the sky a minute, the people around me for a minute, and then back to the sidewalk. I do this until I arrive back home.

• • •

THIS LAST episode is enough reason for me to make arrangements to see my doctor. I will have to go home and stay somewhere, so I call my parents to see if it would be all right to stay with them for a few days.

I haven't talked much about them, but they are a big part of my life. I know this is not the case for every young man, and I realize I've been fortunate enough to have my parents' support, throughout my childhood, my surgery, my high school years, and college career. I don't know if I got my critical thinking skills from them, but as a result of their pushing for the best, it is obvious they instilled in me their drive.

JOSHUA HOLMES

Unlike Michael, I didn't have constant concerns about being a sinner, and going to hell on a regular basis. Yes, I grew up in a religious household, as you may have gathered already in examining my thoughts. And, yes, I had that holy book, The Bible. But as long as I was wise, and made good decisions, I would not have to worry about anything. If I acted irresponsibly, my parents made clear, I would have to reap what I sowed. And this concept applied to me physically and spiritually.

Whereas Michael was threatened, I was encouraged to do the right thing, to live by The Book so that I could enjoy Christianity, and life in general for that matter. For a while they weren't into earrings and tattoos and wild hair, but with time, I can only guess, that changed. I imagine they thought preaching about physical appearance was second to pushing a lifestyle that included God.

As long as I tried to do the latter, I concluded, I was good to go. Even during my brief rebellious streak, when I didn't necessarily like my parents or anything they said, I deep down understood that their approach made sense. Since appearance was rarely an issue, I had no reason to pursue any form of body art. Thus, my current disinterest in permanent ink-jobs and holes in my body, and my incredulity about Michael's recent visit to the tattoo/piercing parlor. So he's in love. Why ruin his body?

Anyway, When I hear my Mom answer the phone, and she tells me she is putting me on speaker-phone so Dad can hear me, I imagine my parents in their piano room surrounded by pictures of jazz musicians playing instruments, next to the Grand, under the winding stairwell that leads to their loft above.

ELECTRIC

"I got a call from the doctor, and he gave me good news. I want to surprise you. Would it be alright if I catch a bus and visited a few days?"

Being the awesome son that I am, they have no problem with that.

• • •

I AM OFF on Fridays, so I schedule a visit to the doctor's office for the end of the week. On Thursday night, I arrive at the State College bus terminal and catch a Greyhound en-route to Harrisburg. The ride is not bad, about two hours.

For the first half hour I look out the bus window. The scenery is just incredible. My surroundings evolve as the thick, colorful woods and foliage bordering the mountain streams thins into flat, more developed land with very little vegetation. Meanwhile, the empty, windy roads turn into heavily traveled highways. Because I'm in the mountains, I enjoy observing the vast changes in climate, and it passes time away.

The time also goes by because I bring the book about the blind mountain climber. After the half hour of observation, I pull the novel from my travel bag. A couple weeks after I first skimmed through the novel at Barnes & Noble, I went back to the bookstore and bought it. Even though I find it difficult reading about the success of others, I get into this book for the remainder of the journey, and, before I know it, I am at the Harrisburg terminal.

My parents warmly greet me after I have gotten situated in their car, a sharp Jaguar. It's so great to see them. We exchange hugs and kisses, and then we settle on a restaurant where we will eat our dinner. We settle on a restaurant called Gullifty's, an interesting place with good food.

In Gullifty's, the eating area is poorly lit, sconces with an orange glow the only source of light. It is smoky, crowded, and loud. Several local bands perform on a stage in the downstairs bar, and it reverberates our booth. The waitresses are often strange, but the menu is great. It keeps us coming back.

After being seated by an eccentric hostess, while waiting for our dinners to arrive, my mother says, "You'll never guess who is working over at the neurology clinic."

"Yeah?" I say. "Who?"

"Mary Grace. You remember her. Right?" I think, *Do I ever!*

In a reserved tone, I say, "Yeah. I remember. She was good to me."

Sitting in the shaky booth, I am happy to be with my parents, and the news about Mary Grace makes it even better.

• • •

WHEN I show at the doctor's office, I walk to the front desk and sign the necessary paperwork, all the confidentiality crap. Handing the information to the secretary, I get sick to my stomach, thinking about my years as a constant patient. I look around. Sitting in the waiting room, other patients who probably know what I am talking about make noises, grunting, sighing, even yelling out, as a few seats away there is a man and woman with extensive neurological damage.

After waiting about a half hour longer than the actual scheduled appointment, I hear the door to the individual, examination rooms open. I hear a woman's voice say, "Chris?" The woman is Mary

GRAND MAL

Grace. She has on a white jacket, and is holding the clipboard with all the information I previously filled out. She is happy to see me, and smiles broadly.

I go through the regular protocol: the measurement of my height, the tracking of my weight. I usually don't care what people think of me, but because Mary Grace is the nurse following through with the protocol, I feel very self-conscious. I mean, I'm not fat or short, but I'm no skinny buff either. Of the two body types, I'd prefer the latter, especially when I am in the presence of someone significant.

She looks great, in my opinion, a sight for sore eyes. *She is definitely the ideal woman for me*, I think; Her long blond hair; her bright blue eyes; her smile; her slender body. She is as nice and wonderful as I recall from our days in high school.

Once we are in the examination room, she takes my blood pressure, which is probably higher because she is there, and she asks me how I've been. With a heavily beating heart, I shyly tell her I am nearing the end of grad school, and she congratulates me. I enjoy her touch on my arm and back, very nice. I ask her how things have been for her, and she tells me she loves being a nurse. Unfortunately, her work comes to a close. She documents my health status, and even though she probably shouldn't, she hugs me goodbye.

I see the doctor afterwards, which is much less exhilarating. I am happy he believes this new medicine will work, and I thankfully and willingly discuss my new options, but I don't enjoy the doctor near as much as the nurse.

• • •

JOSHUA HOLMES

A MONTH HAS passed since I have returned to my apartment at school. Everyday, I can see how in love Michael is. He won't stop talking about Linda! Linda said this. Linda said that. Linda did this. Linda did that. As annoying as it is, I know I'll probably do the same when I find my special someone.

Michael is an entirely different person. And I'm not just referring to his tattoo and earring. It is his overall demeanor; it changes on a whim if Linda wishes. Recently, he told me he has news, and I am curious to know which Michael I'll see then. He said he wants to tell me something over dinner at the cafeteria tonight. Before he does though, he told me he is going to walk Linda home.

I know this will take a while, so I go to the West Commons lobby early to watch some television, a game on the Big Ten Network possibly. There are some wooden benches in front of the TV, but I am uncertain whether or not I want to sit down. The seats are far from comfortable; there aren't any pillows. I don't want to sit if I can't have pillows, right? Right. So I stand. And I enjoy a game until it's time to head upstairs.

On the second floor now, I hand over the ID card I use to buy my meals to the lunch lady at the cafeteria entrance, and then take it back after it has been approved and twelve bucks has come out of my lion cash account. Wincing at the thought of such an amount decreasing my allotted spending, I enter through the door into the stuffy catering establishment.

I do not see Michael. For the moment, I sit down and wait. This place is a mad house! There are five main stations where kids hired

ELECTRIC

by the school serve Chinese food, pizza, burgers and fries, and, my favorite, desserts like cake, cookies, and fresh Creamery ice cream.

• • •

As I wait, I think about the classes that have really helped me understand how people with and without disabilities reason and function. Human behavior intrigues me, and my program has a pretty thorough curriculum that, I think, helps you learn about it. This is what I need and like about the program, the substantial classes.

The Cedar Clinic, where I work for one of these classes, has its downfalls. The place hasn't been upgraded for ages. So, unfortunately, as a result, it is outdated, way too small, and, in my opinion, very uncomfortable.

I occasionally hear professors in my department discuss the impact of budgetary restraints. And at one point, considering the size of the university, I found their concerns hard to believe. But after laboring day and night at the clinic, hearing no mention of future upgrades, my doubts have dissipated, and I now accept a lack of funding is why my training ground isn't up to par.

In the clinic, there are about eight prison cell-like meeting rooms with large one-way mirrors covering the walls. Each room has two chairs in the center. One for the client. One for the counselor. In these cells, some additional décor includes a floor lamp, and a table with flowers, a microphone, a full tissue box for emotional clients, and a phone for emergencies (in case I have a seizure, for instance). Not a whole lot.

JOSHUA HOLMES

At the same time, I have good conversation with colleagues who are equally uncomfortable. As long as we are quiet behind closed doors, we can discuss our work, help each other explore counseling approaches, and refine the wording of our progress notes. And in regards to paperwork, I only have to put the Data Assessment Plans (DAPs) in a manila envelope, and walk down the hall to hand them in to the clinic coordinators. While the environment can be challenging, it has its benefits.

Working with clients in general for my practicum class is about as close for me to being a counselor as it will get at Penn State. This requires dedication to several hours of watching videos on old TVs in a hot, cramped room, and taking notes and completing self-evaluations in another, even smaller room. Depending on the number of referrals, I have carried a caseload of five clients at once.

During my sessions, I give my client direct eye contact. I dress appropriately, in a button-down shirt and slacks, and present myself in a professional manner, monitoring my posture and any non-verbals that might convey negative vibes.

While there is no room for error in this class, after my sessions with certain clients, I feel a sense of accomplishment. I am helping people who are hurting to sort through their problems, and when they have a revelation, or show signs of self-pride as a result of seeing things from multiple perspectives, it is rewarding. I have contributed to their happiness, and I go home happy as well.

• • •

GRAND MAL

JUST AS I am about to reflect on another influential class, Michael walks up behind me, taps me on my left shoulder, and then walks to my right. He does this to me all the time, so I know he is the culprit. Nevertheless, I am glad he is here, because I was about to give up on him.

Above all the chatter and gossip, Michael says, "Whaazuup homie!"

"Yo!" I reply, a bit anxious. "I'm good." I turn around and say with a smile, "So what's the story here, Mike. I've been waiting a while."

"Sorry. Busy with Linda."

"Get some food, meet me back here, and then you can tell me what you want me to know."

"Alright."

• • •

WHEN MICHAEL and I have sat down, we have to speak a little louder. All the undergrads are gossiping about petty things like who dumped who, who has a better haircut, or who got the most drunk the previous night. I still cannot get over how immature these kids are. *I'm sure glad I am not like that*, I think. I cringe when the group behind me erupts, loud streams of laughter filling my ears.

Our conversation begins lively and fun, as always. A lot of kidding and joking. Some light-hearted debate. Soon though, our joking and banter subsides and our discussion becomes sober.

"You know, Chris," Michael says, touching his ear where his highlighter usually resides, "I'm seriously considering dropping out of school." I immediately forget the obnoxious sounds around me. I stare at him in silence, my mouth open for at least three minutes.

"You've got to be kidding me, Michael!" I say. "Why the heck would you do that? You are nuts!" I am irate, shocked beyond measure.

"Cool it, bro. Let me finish," he says defensively, his lip starting to curl, his thick uni-brow starting to furrow. I can sense that the gossipers have turned their heads to listen in, to stare. I calm down and tell him to go on. "I'm in love, man. I don't want this school stuff anymore. I just want to be with Linda, on my own and not on campus."

"Well, I think it's pretty stupid if you want the truth." I am still in awe. "We are almost done here!"

"I thought you, of all people, would understand." He is thoroughly pissed. His voice is starting to rise. The employees at the dessert station now look at us. He pushes back his chair, picks up his tray, none of his food touched. "You know what Chris. I actually don't need your approval! I love her! She's got great parents! And she loves me!" He storms off, and everyone stares me down in a way that suggests they disapprove of me. I can almost hear them thinking, *What a dummy.*

I have a client to see in a few minutes, so I breathe deeply to cool off. I don't want to arrive at the Cedar Clinic disheveled. As I get up, I roll my eyes and think, *Considering the topic, that went pretty well.*

• • •

ELECTRIC

At the moment, despite my earlier, hostile discussion with Michael, things are going well. I just had a female client draw some personal conclusions. It was like a light bulb just lit up in her head. She realized what was holding her back (self-doubt, mostly), and how much power she has over her future. The first step to recovery.

Back in my room, I am rehearsing my introduction and confidentiality statement I have to reiterate with every new client. "As you know . . . everything we talk about stays in the counseling room unless I sense that you are going to hurt yourself or someone else . . . a child or an elderly adult." And the most embarrassing part. "And I have to tell you that I do have seizures. Are you uncomfortable with that?"

I am pondering over the last part when I hear the phone ring. I stop my rehearsal and think, *It's probably Mom and Dad checking to see how my day went.* To my surprise, it is Mary Grace. Having seen her recently, I have a renewed vision of her. And I like it.

"Hello?" I say, smiling to myself before she even responds.

"Hey Chris. It's Mary Grace." *Oh, cool*, I think.

"I know who it is. You didn't even have to say so." She laughs, and I see her in the doctor's office, in her white jacket, covering her mouth to maintain her professionalism.

"Well. Just calling to let you know the doctor talked to your insurance company, and you are good to go," she says. "You should be able to get your new med at the pharmacy now." It then gets quiet. As I told you earlier, I hate silence.

"You know Mary Grace . . ." More silence. "It was great seeing you again."

JOSHUA HOLMES

"Oh yeah." She says, a different tone in her voice. "Definitely. You too." I hear a chair squeak over the phone. Am I making her nervous? Is she looking around to see if her co-workers are watching? Or, probably the most likely answer, reaching for my records in the nearby file cabinet?

"Well," I say. "Thanks for the call. Talk to you later?"

"Yes. Will do."

• • •

About a week after Michael and I have our confrontational dinner, the Dave Matthews Band comes to town. Following our earlier discussion about my catching a ride with Linda and him to the concert, I reconsidered, and I am currently heading up Bigler Road by myself, a shortcut to the Bryce Jordan Center.

In my opinion, the Bryce Jordan Center is a great place to host special events. It is large and spacious, the round shape of the white structure conducive to large crowds. Inside, various vendors sell food at concession stands. Other vendors sell merchandise for the performing bands. And the atrium that circles out around the seating area is big enough so you can make it to your section in a timely manner.

Blue-collar families and students alike come together to share an entertaining evening at one of the best venues in all of Centre County. I get thrills just thinking about my time there. I don't know. I guess it's great for me because I am around a lot of different people again. Kind of like at the HUB and at Beaver Stadium.

GRAND MAL

Before I know it, I am close to the entrance. I am shivering because, no matter the season, the area just outside the Center remains chilly. A dry breeze just sucks the air out of me. Fortunately, I don't have to endure the chill too long, for the line to get inside moves quickly.

At the entrance, a security guard approaches me and says, "Spread your legs and raise your arms."

• • •

AFTER PASSING the security point, I hand my ticket to a lady dressed in a white, button down shirt, black slacks, a formal black vest, and a red bowtie. She tears off the stub, and hands the other half of the ticket back to me. She tells me to enjoy the show, and I tell her to have a good evening.

Inside the atrium, I buy some popcorn and a Pepsi, and then walk down to my seat. The Center is packed. I trip over a few people in the process of getting to my seat, but I get there and situate myself in a way so that I can place my food and drink out of harm's way.

There is a man in front of me, dressed in a tie-dye shirt (similar to Sam's) that says 'Legalize Hemp'. He has a long mullet and spectacles comparable to those worn by John Lennon. He leans back in my direction and says with a toothless smirk, "I've seen these guys five times! Gone to 'most every concert! You?" His breath reeks of alcohol. He is clearly intoxicated, and I am not interested in speaking with him. He looks at me, pushes a doobie in his mouth, and waits for a response.

JOSHUA HOLMES

I act as if I didn't hear him, turn away and pick up my soda. I know the types of people who can come to see the Dave Matthews Band. There are the social weed smokers, the druggies, and the deadheads. Mr. Mullet seems to be a drunk deadhead. I'm not saying there aren't classy people who come to the Bryce Jordan Center for some contemporary jazz, but the carefree nature of the music, and the lyrics about the joys of getting high often brings out the craziest of people (not to mention a select few who enjoy surfing the crowds, exposing their nude bodies to the world). I smile at this thought, as I remember when it happened a few years back at the Hershey Park stadium.

The concert hasn't even begun, but the air is thick with smoke; the illegal drug a dark fog floating around me. It is stuffy, and the fog makes me claustrophobic, but I have gone through this before. I know what the concerts are like. I have been to six of them. My favorite band's gigs have always made my claustrophobia go away. For an hour and a half, I wait for Dave, Leroi, Boyd, Carter, and Stefan to walk on stage. I am surprised the ushers haven't approached Mr. Mullet.

• • •

WHEN THE lights dim, the vapor seems to fade. The crowd roars. In the dark, we all hear the smooth saxophone sound. The bass guitar follows a short, horn solo. Still in the black, the violin and drums come to life. And finally, I recognize Dave Matthews is strumming his acoustic guitar. In unison, they open the concert

ELECTRIC

with their famous song, 'Crash'. The moment Dave begins to sing, the stage lights flash on, and the crowd roars even louder.

On either side of me, young couples are kissing, hugging, and dancing with one another. All around, other people in the audience are holding up cigarette lighters, giving a candlelight ceremony effect.

I begin to sing, "I'll be your Dixie chicken if you'll be my Tennessee lamb, and we can walk together down in Dixieland. Crash into me." A girl behind me rubs my shoulders, and I look back thinking, *What the heck?* She is wearing a bandanna over dark French braided hair, a halter-top, and very short shorts. She says, "Crash into me, baby." And she sticks out her tongue. I shake my head, and turn around. First it was Mr. Mullet, and now The Tongue. What an experience.

Again, though, Dave and the band overwhelm me, and I continue to have a great time. They start to jam, which they have long been known for, and their ability to improvise their songs on a whim is unbelievable. The keyboardist starts playing a cover band song, 'Super Freak', and they all join in with their individual instruments to build the crescendo.

Leroi, the saxophonist, is a big guy who plays with sunglasses and a straight face. Carter on the other hand drums with a big smile on his face. Boyd is constantly sliding his rod over the violin strings; his eyebrows lifted high, his smile spread wide. Dave and Stefan sing and play with intensity, and dance while they perform, moving their feet back and forth.

At the peak of the song, the strobes start to sparkle. Green, red, and blue lights flicker on and off with each beat. The colorful display continues for a long time, and the music overwhelms me, filling me with that happiness I feel at the football games. The display grows more and more elaborate, like fireworks during a celebration, until the song slows down and eventually comes to a close.

I stand for three hours as they play old and new tunes, and Mr. Mullet and The Tongue leave me be. I haven't stood for three hours straight since football season, but I'm running on adrenaline. I am at Penn State, taking a break from my work, listening to my all-time, favorite band while feasting on junk food. It doesn't get much better than this. The air is thicker with smoke now, but I am used to it. I knew I would get over it, and time passes quickly. I tap my fingers on the back of the chair in front of me, and sway to the music.

Before I know it, the concert is over, and it is time to stop dancing. Dave and the band close with their usual song, 'Stay', and he thanks everyone for coming out. He says, "See you all next year. Be good to one another, you hear?" And the stage goes dark.

I think, *Man! Once again, they surpassed my expectations!*

• • •

WALKING HOME, I think about Michael and Linda; whether or not they enjoyed the music or made out the whole time like the other couples around me. I wonder what my night with them would have been like. I didn't have a seizure, a stoned deadhead said hello, and a girl hit on me. Not that that's a bad thing. I just wasn't hanging with friends. For a moment, the thought makes me angry. But I again tell myself I am being unreasonable.

GRAND MAL

If I were to ask Michael and Linda about it, they both might get defensive. Unfortunately, I tend to ask questions in the wrong way. I am often misunderstood. I inquire about things most people don't like to discuss. It's not my fault I want to find explanations.

Speaking of finding things, I sometimes have difficulty finding my way home in the dark. I have to ask people where to go. Tonight, though, I know where I am. I cross University Drive, which is barricaded, pass the Bursars Office to my left, as well as the Wagner Building (a.k.a. the ROTC building). Orange cones and orange netting line the sidewalks to protect the kids from hazardous areas under construction. So many students are walking home to their dorms.

I, on the other hand, am going to White Course. So I stroll beyond all the dorms. I head towards the enormous walkway crossing North Atherton Road, where Michael claimed he wasn't winded from the hike. I won't deny it, tonight. I am exhausted. And I have to get up early tomorrow for my individual supervision meeting concerning my clients at the Cedar Clinic.

When I reach my apartment, I might read a while to settle myself down, to clear my head of all the sights and sounds of the concert. I will not watch TV, though. I'll have a chance to do that just after daybreak, as it is protocol to view a video of my counseling session with my supervisor.

• • •

I DO READ when I get home, but I fail to notice that the red light on my phone is flashing, that I obviously have a new message.

JOSHUA HOLMES

I accidentally close my eyes, and doze off on my bed with my glasses on. And as with the lights from the ambulance at the game, the flashing light on my phone throws me into a seizure. Right now, the intensity of my seizure is pulsating.

Because I just went to the Dave Matthews Band concert, my mind is filled to the brim with images of dancers, singers, instrumentalists, and lovers. Not to mention visuals of the entire auditorium blanketed with a suffocating cloud of weed and apparitions holding lighters in the air. These are normal images, but I am about to see a distorted version of them I wouldn't wish on anyone.

My brain currents are presently at full throttle, and I am heading into a delusional state. In this state, I am entering the Bryce Jordan Center again, falling soon after, and hitting my head. I am sweating from my efforts to breath, and I silently cry. My lifeless body is pinned under the Center's smoky coating. I can't lift my head, move my arms or legs, or make the dancers and singers aware of my horrible condition. Like a fireworks display gone awry, the stage lights are intensely flashing in my face every color imaginable.

When those people nearby do see me, they all laugh. Mr. Mullet scoffs, says, "Look at him. It is his fault he hurt himself. He shouldn't have been tapping his fingers on my chair!!" I begin to wail. I want to say, "Get away from me!" But all I can do is loudly grunt and attempt to grab at the air. I am so scared.

The Tongue bends over me, and says, "Yeah. He wouldn't be my Dixie Chicken either!" I see ushers with small bodies and big heads running down the stairs to my aisle. Behind them, I see Dave,

ELECTRIC

Leroi, Stefan, Carter, and Boyd making faces at me. Then they laugh and laugh and laugh. My favorite band. All of them making fun of me.

My dream is torture. My sleep is torture. My seizure is torture.

• • •

MY RESTLESSNESS makes getting up less torturous, though. Remember Mrs. Patterson? The sometimes aggressive, but mostly caring, bouncy-haired professor with whom I had difficulty my first semester? In my second year, she is my practicum supervisor. We get along well now, and I don't have to worry about her piercing eyes boring into me near as much.

When I arrive at Mrs. Patterson's office, I can see from the hall that she is moving a few pieces of paper (Imagine! Only three papers!) off of her file cabinets, putting them on her empty desk so that the television and cassette player will fit on top of the metal surface.

I tap on the door, which is only half open, and she tells me to come in. I sit in that once dreaded seat. It isn't quite as scary as it used to be. It helps that I'm tired, and that sitting in any chair sounds good to me.

After Mrs. Patterson inserts the cassette, she soberly asks me what I thought about my session with my client.

"I think it really went well," I say with a nod. "Really well."

On the television, I look so much more reserved than I feel. I have my legs tucked under my seat because I really want to bounce my foot when speaking with my client, and I have my hands folded because I know I will start tapping my shoes if I don't. Yet it all looks so natural!

My questions don't sound near as bad as I thought, either. My client's reactions are very positive. Everything about the session makes me feel better about myself. I might just turn out to be a good counselor!

When we are done watching the video, Mrs. Patterson wipes a few dust particles that fall out of the cassette player (no kidding), and then we discuss the plan for my next session. She advises me not to problem solve, but rather let the client take the session where he wants it to go. I assure her I will, and she says, "You've come a long way."

• • •

I GUESS I have come a long way. I'm proud of myself! My hard work is paying off. But I don't know if I can say the same thing about my best friend. Michael has gone somewhere, too, but not in the same way. His Dad's training has disintegrated. Michael has almost stopped working on his homework all together, and he has stopped participating in his debate club.

John and Alex are standing outside my apartment door to see if Michael and Linda are ready for a debate. Both Michael and Linda are out and Michael recently told me he was going to quit the group meetings. Alex's forehead is creased like you wouldn't believe, and his pudgy fingers are in the air, just emphasizing something I didn't hear. John's forehead has a nice white highlight in which I can see a

GRAND MAL

distorted version of myself (when he comes to a momentary standstill, that is), and he is annoyed that I didn't open the door sooner.

I don't want to tell them that their intellectual colleagues have no desire to participate in their explorations of philosophy any longer, yet I have to say something. I don't want them to feel rejected as I frequently did growing up, so I say, "Guys, I'm sorry to break the bad news, but Michael and Linda will be busy with other things from now on."

I imagine how much John and Alex will miss their weekly gatherings around that pitiful table, the camaraderie and banter as they tried to get comfortable on the hard seats. Yeah, they will have a hard time walking away from the experience.

It was a time when Alex could let off steam about his nasty and neglectful Grandparents, and express his desire for a Dad, a "real" role model. This time also allowed John to stay in the present, without worries of being attacked.

While I did not really enjoy the banter, I enjoyed some of the theory, and was learning more about how my friends, yes, my friends now, thought. I will miss the experience, too. If for no other reason, I was becoming more open to new ideas. I now know that it is important to listen, even if I disagree, and this philosophy falls in line with that of my counseling program.

"What?" they say simultaneously. "How can that be true?"

"They are finished with the club." They turn to leave, shaking their heads.

"I know," I agree, shaking my own head. "It's sad."

JOSHUA HOLMES

• • •

To MY dismay, I am not aware of the moving date, when Michael has to be out of his room. So, initially, I am annoyed. And, to top it off, I still do not approve of his decision to leave school. But again, my opinion doesn't mean much at this point.

Michael and Linda start cleaning early in the morning, too early for me, and I do not know why they can't wait. I hear a familiar sound, the large golden dolly from the community center vestibule crashing against the sides of the doorway. Once in our kitchen, the squeaky wheels screech to a halt, and, still in bed, I say to myself, "For crying out loud. Am I ever going to get a solid sleep?"

Perhaps when I graduate, when I'm too tired to do anything but close my eyes! I guess I'll find out when I get there. In the meantime, I know complaining isn't going to put me back to sleep. So I get up. I recognize that I will be better off getting my endorphins going. Once again, in my classic Christopher fashion, I dunk my head in the sink and push my matted hair back into an acceptable position. "Morning," I say to the busy couple, yawning. "You really know how to give a nice wake up call."

"Sorry, Chris," Linda says, peeking from behind Michael. *What's up with all this peeking?* I think. *Are we playing hide and seek here?*

"It's alright," I lie. "So where do we begin?"

"Well you could help us with the boxes. They need folded and taped so we can start putting my things inside." Michael points to the boxes in the corner, and hands me the tape. The boxes are right next to my art supplies. "You might want to brush your teeth, too. I don't want you to knock us out on moving day!" We laugh a little,

ELECTRIC

which is a nice change from the yelling he gave me before the Dave Matthews Band concert.

The living room is bright today; the blinds pulled all the way up. The sun is shining, and I have to squint for a while. I think about the night Michael and I stood before the same window talking about the pitiful ditch by the bus stop. It really wasn't all that long ago. I think about doing our homework in silence, and throwing the foam football around while watching the Steelers.

I then think about the day Michael first brought Linda to our apartment, how the door was locked. And when he smirked those goofy smirks while cooking for her. When she walked out of his room in a nighty, my hair a crazy mess.

"Are you going to be taking the television, Michael?" I ask, hoping he won't.

"I'd like to," he replies, itching his ear. "Are you all right with that? Because I was going to pay you the amount you put towards it." While it is hard to part with such a nice piece of technology, I am okay with it. I have a television in my room.

"Yeah," I say. "That'll work."

Before we start carrying the boxes down to a rented truck, I go to the bathroom and thoroughly scrub my teeth. While I had the urge to make my friend suffer a whiff, a sign of a true friend, I have mercy on him. No use leaving a sour taste in his mouth.

It takes several trips up and down the elevator to finish the move. And the move leaves its mark. That's for sure. The dolly has destroyed my doorway, the doorframe nicked and sliced, and I can pretty much forget getting back my initial down payment. Very disappointing.

Even more disappointing, though, is the fact that my best friend will be gone at the end of the day. For good? I don't know. I hope not. But things don't look too promising. Michael just told me he'll be proposing very soon. A good indicator.

Let me clarify, though, that I feel the time I spent alone helped me grow. I'm more independent. At one point, I needed Michael by my side just to get by. No longer. I will remain friends with John and Alex. I will continue going to karate. I'll deal with my Epilepsy with assistance from above, and I'll finish up my degree a stronger person.

After I put the last box away in the back of the truck, I turn to Michael and Linda. I hug them, and look at Michael. "I'm going to miss you."

"Yeah. Well don't get all sappy," he says, patting me on the back. "We'll be around."

• • •

PART FOUR:

SPRING AND SUMMER SEMESTER, SEASON FINALE

I DECIDE NOT to get emotional about Michael and Linda's departure. My emotions have to be saved for other things. After all, I have an internship to get ready for. Perhaps one at the Office of Rehabilitation Therapy, the agency my department wants every student to get into so they can maintain their almost 100 percent job placement success rate.

I have to make the calls to all the ORT county administrators in the state for possible interviews, the calls to Pennsylvania's Civil Service office so I'm on "The List". The list that supposedly helps me and tells each county I'm available for a position. The list that can, I've heard, also come back to bite me in the rear. The list some administrators can tell me I'm not on if I have a disability like Epilepsy, even if I am.

Do I settle for an unpaid internship with mentoring responsibilities at a smaller agency, or work for a possibly discriminatory government agency counseling, shuffling papers, and pushing as many people as likely into employment? A tough question that is emotionally challenging.

So I have other things than my friend leaving to think about. I'm putting all options on the table. And I'll see soon what happens.

• • •

THE SPRING semester is moving along slowly, because ORT has bitten me in the rear over and over and over again, just as predicted. And sure enough, my transportation problem has provided the state agency an excuse to eliminate any professional opportunities I have earned.

I have gone to ten different interviews, all of which I did well, and been turned down. Talk about a major blow to my ego, and an incredibly disheartening series of events. By now, all my friends from the original group are gone, either in their internship or working full-time. And I am still waiting with no opportunities in sight.

I call my parents every night to vent. I sort of feel bad about it. They shouldn't have to worry about me after a hard day's work. They have their own issues to deal with. Who else do I have to talk to, though? Well, I guess there is Sam. Yeah. Now that I think about it, I do have Sam.

• • •

ELECTRIC

"OK SAM. So here's the deal," I say. "I'm still unemployed with no sign of anything in sight. And I am stressing like you wouldn't believe."

"You know, Chris. Don't be in such a hurry. Waiting isn't such a bad thing."

Observing the new pictures on the walls in the bookstore, and then the new bookshelves to be filled, I say, "That's easy for you to say."

Staring at me intensely, he replies, "I'm an old man, chap. Look at me. I lost a wife ages ago over money. I longed for but never had a son. I have a bum leg. And dreads that look a hundred years old. Don't tell me I don't know about time."

This shuts me up. He's right. "Sorry."

"It's fine. Just remember that patience is a virtue." Cliché, but true I guess. And then a broad smile crosses his face. "On a different topic. I've noticed that you have been keeping an eye on the artwork on my walls. I know you are a great artist and I think it's about time you give a show."

"Oh, Sam. Would you let me?" I look at the pictures again, more intensely. I am trying to visualize my drawings in certain positions along the wall. The mildewy smell of used books and the odor of coffee wafting from a nearby table does not distract me. I'm too excited by the thought of my own show.

Smiling what feels like an evil smile, he says, "In time, son. Very soon that wall will be yours to use."

I pick up a book and purchase it. *In time*, I think. *Very funny.*

• • •

JOSHUA HOLMES

I TAKE THE book I bought at Webster's to a secret garden I found in front of the Alumni Hall just recently. The garden is hidden behind a white gazebo wrapped in the brown and maroon leaves of two Japanese Maples. A narrow pathway covered in silt opens into a shady area with wraparound benches. Ready for a nice read, I take a seat and cross my legs. At my feet, several slate stones accentuate a small, man-made pond where tiny ducklings float on the surface and a turtle's head peeks through the water ripples. This little world is so beautiful it is surreal, and a place so remote I could stay here forever.

Reading forever. Huh. That's a thought. And it's not like I don't have the time. Yeah, I have some papers to write for a few classes, but other than that . . . Nothing but time. Just waiting for an internship opportunity to hop on.

Since the nonfiction novel about the blind mountain climber was good, I bought another nonfiction novel; only this one is about a guy with quadriplegia who paints with his mouth. The story is right up there with the story of an artist/novelist with severe Cerebral Palsy who goes from poor boy to nationally acclaimed painter and author in *My Left Foot*.

I look at my left foot. It makes me think about my karate class, how much I have improved. How my body is doing more than I ever thought possible. And how, surprisingly, I am seizing less. I will be learning new kicking techniques this week. I have been kicking punching bags that my opponent holds up, but from what I understand, I will be kicking my opponents without punching bags, and

GRAND MAL

with very little protection; maybe gloves and a mask at most. This thought peps me up.

A nice breeze cools my warm hands, and the book's pages between my fingers rustle quietly. I hear a splash in the water, and I assume the turtle is ducking beneath the surface. While I could stay here for many more hours, I fold the corner of the last page I've read, close my book, and bow out of the secret garden, back into the real world.

• • •

IN THE real world I have spent a lot of time focusing on the inconvenience of my seizures, and of waiting. I haven't focused on one positive thing. Ever since I started taking the new medicine, my seizures have decreased substantially. And my visit to the neurologist, and correspondence with Mary Grace, has led to a less distracting lifestyle. These are good things. Necessary things, in my opinion. Why, you ask? Because I don't know if I could take unemployment and constant seizing at once. It just might break my will.

Despite yelling at God, at my lowest moment He opened a door and made His presence so clear. He had the woman I've had a crush on my entire life take care of my prescriptions. Too coincidental to be fate. I haven't been given more than I can handle. Given enough, though, that my "human resiliency", a term frequently used in the counseling field, was and continues to be necessary. I persist in hopes that He will shine through.

JOSHUA HOLMES

For some reason, as I walk past the Alumni Hall, approach Pollock Road, and the garden disappears, I feel rejuvenated. I sense that there is something good on the horizon.

• • •

MY PREMONITION may prove true today, twenty-four hours after I have visited the garden. My internship woes could be wiped away. Just recently, I called a friend of my advisor's, a doctor currently working as a counselor at a job placement agency called CareerForce. Over the phone, she said she would give me an internship if I give her a good interview.

So I am walking up Allen Street at the moment. I am dressed in a powder blue button-down shirt, a navy suit coat, navy slacks, and a navy blue and powder blue striped tie. My Adam's apple is bulging out of my neck, which is a bit uncomfortable, but other than that, I feel great. My head is held high, my dark hair slicked back. I take a deep breath, and I smell my cologne, my skin exuding a nice aroma.

I look at my reflection in the windows of the surrounding stores to make sure I look handsome, and I smile, giving myself a thumbs up. I am almost at Panera Bread, where I made arrangements to meet with the doctor. Just above my cologne, I can smell sandwiches and soup, a great combination.

The doctor told me she would be in a plaid shirt and pants, that her hair is short and dark. I see so many women with dark hair sitting at small tables, circular booths, and couches. While I am excited, I momentarily get worried. What if I don't find her? But my concerns go away when I see a lady in the corner wave at me. She

ELECTRIC

is wearing an open, black sweater over her plaid button-down. No wonder I missed her!

I walk over to her and stick my hand out for a shake. "Hello Dr. Webber. I am Chris."

• • •

I HAVE ALMOST every interview question and response out there memorized. As I sit down, I quietly recite my opening, and hope for easy queries. My heart is beating fast, and I am shaking inside. When the questions are basic, mainly pertaining to my counseling experience, and the requirements to fulfill my internship, I relax.

However, I must say the lack of affect in her voice confuses me. Is she bored? Am I coming across confident enough? An hour passes, and as the clock ticks, I overcome my self-doubt and make an assumption; that she senses I am reliable. And before I know it, Dr. Webber says, "As far as I'm concerned, you can start tomorrow."

I say, "Dr. Webber, thank you so much. You have no idea how grateful I am."

"No problem," she replies, smiling. "You should have called me sooner!"

• • •

WHEN I step into the CareerForce office for the first time, I am so pleased. It is quiet, open and airy, a pleasant atmosphere. Every employee is talking softly either in their cubicles, near the printer, or at the front desk. Each one seems to be enjoying their colleague's company and assistance. Some of them stop what they are doing to welcome me, and I tell them a little bit about myself, to break the ice.

When they all hear that I am completing my master's degree at Penn State, they congratulate me, and I smile appreciatively. I especially enjoy the secretaries. They seem as if they were born to meet and greet.

One secretary in particular, Sally her name is, reminds me of Jenny on *Forrest Gump*, the blond hippy in a long dress who carried a guitar around after joining the Black Panthers. While Sally isn't a Black Panther member and isn't carrying a guitar, she does have Jenny's golden eyes, a plain, full-length dress, and loose, scraggly hair held in place by a red bandanna. Her voice is so fluid, and she pats my back when she says she looks forward to working with me.

Dr. Webber says, "Well, Chris. Now that you have met some of the employees, I'll show you around, and then we can talk some more."

In the front area, there are about twelve computer terminals for unemployed individuals to job search. The people sitting before the keyboards are unkempt, dressed in torn clothing and covered in long, ratty hair. All their faces are tense as they concentrate on the agency's database. And they seem to know what they are doing, almost as if they visit the office regularly.

Dr. Webber walks me down a hall. She walks with intensity, as if she's on a mission. To some extent, she is. I can tell she is excited, but she maintains a solemn expression. She is kind but serious. I later learn that this is just her personality.

She points to a room on my left with more computers, where I assume the career counselors teach certain classes. Just opposite the computer room is a large conference room. Any number of meetings could be held here. Moving on, she points to three small rooms that all contain a tiny table, a chair, and a phone. She says, "Customers who need to make cold calls to employers can use these rooms."

The tour continues, and even though I've been in several offices, I'm still interested. After all, I'll be working here for the next three months. So, I am best off learning my way around immediately. Dr. Webber briefly shows me the last conference room, the bathroom location, and the small kitchen/eating area. In the corner of the eating area, I see a candy machine, where I can buy candy for a quarter. I smile and think, *Yes!*

Dr. Webber must sense my delight, for she adds, "By the way, there's a vending machine around the corner." I think, *Yes, Yes, Yes!*

• • •

STANDING WITH my student clients at Penn Tech, I say, "Yes. I think you will do well if you come here for school." Dr. Webber nods in agreement, a slight smile on her face. The technical school is small in comparison to Penn State University, but I have never seen a technical school so nice and spread out. In my opinion, the layout is impressive. Perfect for students who have adjustment issues. The college does not have numerous dorms that take up space, but rather a few apartment complexes that house everyone on campus. We all begin towards one of the complexes.

"Maybe," one of the older girls says. Jane, a chubby redhead with hazel eyes and bad teeth, is challenged both mentally and physically. She has depression, and walks with a limp; her demeanor always solemn, her one leg pretty atrophied. Her condition has prevented

JOSHUA HOLMES

her from excelling in high school, which is why she was referred to Dr. Webber's program. She might have some impairments, but I believe she has real potential. "Maybe not," she adds.

While I believe in her, I have to be realistic too. She has multiple hurdles to jump over in order to reach some form of success, of normalcy or independence. Unlike other students her age, Jane will have to work twice as hard to achieve half of what "ordinary" kids are capable of; any chance of social play limited just to keep up academically. As you may have gathered by now, I'm an exception to the rule. And for all I know, she could be too.

The entrance to the complex is rustic, long shadows extending from a red, brick archway with an open black, cast iron fence. I feel like I am at a baseball game, ready to hand in a ticket so I can go inside to find my seat. I even have to walk by a nice patch of green grass with four white stones at the patches' edges that could pass for bases.

I walk in last place; behind the students who are absorbed by the information the tour guide is giving us. While I am excited for the students, I again think of the time Michael and I took the tour. We were absorbed, and had high hopes, yet it wasn't enough for my friend. I hope my clients' interest is an indicator of an uninterrupted, bright educational future.

The apartment setup is different but nice. Two students to a bedroom. Of course, I like my apartment better, but that's just me. The parents of the other students on the tour are absolutely thrilled for their sons and daughters who plan to attend in a few months. It

ELECTRIC

is a day of bonding. And to think a prospective bedroom could bring a family together.

I feel as if this trip has improved my relationships with my clients. I think speaking to them all on their level gets rid of the intimidation factor. Yeah. I remember when I thought some of my teachers in school were arrogant, and I don't want to come across that way now.

Jerry, a young man of sixteen with blonde hair, brown eyes, and multiple piercings in the ears digs his hands deep in his pockets, sags his shoulders in despair, and says, "I dunno man. I want to do it. I been accepted, but I failed 'da test.'" Jerry has a learning disability. He comes from a low-income family, and he hasn't been encouraged all that much. I know he can get through this school with a lot of tutoring, and I plan on pushing him hard, going the extra mile to motivate him.

I don't plan to push him too hard, however, for I know what it is like to have others encourage me with good intent, but not acknowledge the impact a condition can have on my ability to perform. I understand how frustrating it can be, and I won't excessively nag him about what I think he can do, if he doesn't believe it himself. Subtlety is key, and I can counsel him in this manner.

I have been doing this for two months now, counseling several students like Jane and Jerry. I enjoy working with the lost youth as opposed to the stubborn college students I probed in my practicum, and I hope, one day, to find a job in youth counseling.

• • •

JOSHUA HOLMES

THINKING ABOUT my hopes for a job in this field back at my apartment one night, I say a silent prayer, asking for a job opportunity. He gave me my internship; now I need employment.

I sit on the couch in the stillness after talking to God, and look at the wall. Against the wall, there is a box in which I see a rolled up piece of paper bent at the edges. I am curious as to what it is, and I get up to retrieve it.

To my surprise, the decrepit piece of paper holds the picture Michael drew for me when we were boys, the picture of Mary Grace in the color blue, the angel flying in a navy sky, descending into cobalt clouds. What a shock. I look at it, drifting off to a distant place when life was simple. All those memories.

I am so pleased that I have something that I can hold onto, something that reminds me of Michael. I look at it for a while longer, soaking up the distorted image of my favorite nurse. His depiction of her is classic. Just awesome.

I place the drawing in my lap and close my eyes again. I let my worries about finding a permanent job leave my mind, leave them to God, and I turn my thoughts towards graduation. I'm unsure about many things in my future, but I am certain that He will take care of them, and that I want Michael and Mary Grace at my commencement.

• • •

IT IS early at the office, and nobody in the resource area has come to me for assistance on the computers, so I am looking at a letter the Jostens Company recently sent me. The letter is a reminder that

GRAND MAL

commencement is drawing near, and it is about time that I buy graduation announcements, custom seal note cards, and certificates of appreciation as the momentous day approaches.

I am counting the number of weeks I have left of my internship at CareerForce when a heavyset middle-aged lady with premature wrinkles, a bulbous nose, and a big gap between her two front teeth walks up to my desk.

"Ya work 'ere?" I nod and think, *As an intern anyway*. I started not too long ago in the computer area, but I have taken over many of the customer service responsibilities. It's been interesting.

"Yeah. How can I help you?" On the form she hands me, I see her name is Barbie. Let me tell you. This lady looks nothing like Mattel's famous doll.

"Well. I jus' quit my job. The boss was a bastard." *Oh. Good excuse*, I think.

"So what field are you interested in?" I hope she has a special interest, but I don't expect it, as so many that have come in just want money, no matter the source or at what cost.

Barbie laughs nervously, her crow's feet extended in every direction. "I'm desperate, son. Anything will work really."

Inside, I wish now that Sally, the secretary, had a guitar, and would entertain this woman. I have no problem with helping Barbie, but considering Sally is around her age, grew up in her era, and has been in customer service a lot longer, both ladies would bond more quickly, I'm sure. Barbie would listen to Sally.

I try not to push the issue, but I tell Barbie it is important to find a job that best suits her as a person, that it will make the job search process easier if she knows what area of work she wants to pursue, and if she has some realistic goals. I add, "Think about it a minute, and then come get me." She nods.

Back at my desk, I stare at my letter again. I mutter, "A few more weeks, Chris. You can do it." And I will. But as long as I'm at Career-Force, I will continue to do what I love. I will help people match skills to professions, and visit the vending machine in my spare time.

• • •

WEEKS AFTER I have completed my internship, I bring several of my pastel drawings to Webster's bookstore. Sam welcomes me with open arms. "Hello my friend," he says. "You have been patient and your day has come!" He means that today is the day I am going to set up for my art show.

"Thanks Sam."

I go over to the empty walls that are filled with nail holes, put my paintings on a coffee table, and I pull up a chair so I can reach the high places. One by one, I grab my drawings and carefully hang them in a fashion I feel is appropriate. Remembering some material learned in art classes, I attempt to apply certain aesthetic principles, so that the arrangement will pop out, encouraging observers to look more closely.

One of the main reasons I want to showcase my work is to build a reputation, for exposure. And as seen at the Arts Fest, exposure leads to bigger venues, and greater chances of selling some things. To some degree, it is about making money.

ELECTRIC

But even if this is the only show I have, it is a self-esteem builder. It is so satisfying. In the past three years, I have seen that all my practice at Old Main has led to drastic improvements in the quality of my artwork. My eye is catching the tiny details, the power of color experimentation and linear acuity.

I struggle to maintain my balance when hanging my work, but I eventually succeed. Once I have jumped off the chair, I walk to the back of the room. I have some drawings at eye level, my Joe Paterno portraits, some above, just general football drawings, and some below, more portraits, one of which is of my angelic Mary Grace. When I finish examining the layout of my work, I conclude that everything is perfect.

Sam walks to the back of the room too, stands right next to me. He nods, I hope, in approval. I smirk. I can't help it. I mean I just can't wait for everyone to see this!

• • •

"Hey Dr. Webber," I say over the phone the following day. "How are you doing?" When she replies, she is as animated as when I worked with her at CareerForce. Which would mean hardly at all. "Well. Hello Chris. What can I do for you?"

"I was just wondering if you'd like to bring some of the kids to an art exhibit this week. I'm displaying my artwork at Webster's bookstore. Somehow tie the trip to the vocational material in your curriculum."

JOSHUA HOLMES

She sighs. "I was actually just thinking about my plan for the day. You know the summer program is over, but I think Jane and Jerry would enjoy that. Do you think we could make the visit today?"

"Anytime today."

"Wonderful."

In the afternoon, Dr. Webber walks into the bookstore. In a pair of slacks and a different plaid, button-down shirt, she approaches me, greets me, and pats me on the back. "Good to see you, Chris."

"You too." I look past Dr. Webber, and see Jerry and Jane standing there. I am excited to see them, but, like many teens, they aren't enthusiastic about our reunion. Their shoulders sag, and their hellos are half-hearted. "Well," I continue. "Come in and I'll show you my stuff."

The bookstore is small, so the tour is brief, but I spend some time explaining my techniques and the process of painting a portrait. I do it in a way that is easy for Jerry and Jane to grasp, and explain to them that you can find jobs that allow you to use my techniques.

After I'm done, I let them look some more. I stand back, and just watch them. They seem very interested, and it really makes me feel good. Except for the day we visited Penn Tech, I rarely saw the students actively participate in the activities, so their positive reactions to my paintings are a welcome surprise.

When they finish observing everything, Jerry walks and Jane limps to the café, and they both buy drinks from Sam. Dr. Webber follows after them, thanks me, compliments me, and bids me farewell.

GRAND MAL

I don't receive any compliments the rest of the week, but this is fine. I know I'm a decent artist. It is nice to hear that people enjoy realism over the abstract, however I really don't need the affirmation. I'm content with my work, and that's what matters, right?

• • •

THE LAST night of my show, it dawns on me that I should invite Alex and Sam to my graduation. In talking to Sam before I left the bookstore, my trusted mentor said, "You know, I always wanted to father a son from start to finish. You've been that son, but now you're leaving. Now I have to find someone else." Alex has been a friend who always wanted a real father figure. It only makes sense to me that I introduce the two at the ceremony, so that both men might have their dreams fulfilled.

It also dawns on me that perhaps John would benefit from meeting my practicum supervisor, Mrs. Patterson. His negative feelings about teachers might change, if he sees that he can connect on a personal level with a professor, and live without fear of repercussions.

Excited, I spend the rest of the night making calls and presenting invitations. All of the invites accept, and, while it makes me very happy that they are coming, I get a little nervous, too. In a good way.

My final call is the most significant to me. I am again going to talk to Mary Grace. If she could make it to the graduation ceremony, she would make up for Michael's absence tenfold. What could be better than to have my dear angel present during my day of celebration? I think, *Nothing*, as I dial her number.

JOSHUA HOLMES

After three rings, I hear Mary Grace's voice. "Hello?" Man, is it a sweet voice!

"Hey Mary Grace. It's Chris."

"Oh, hi Chris. This is a surprise."

"I hope I'm not calling too late."

"No. Not yet. Getting ready to go to bed, but not yet." I imagine her sitting at the edge of her bed, delicately combing her long hair.

"I don't want to keep you, but I was just calling to see if you'd be interested in coming to my graduation tomorrow. Admission and seating is free." I think, *Please say yes. Please say yes.*

"Well. Thank you for asking, and I'd love to, but I can't promise anything." I hear her mattress squeak. "I mean . . . I don't know if I'll be called into work."

"Just thought I'd invite you. It would be great to see you again."

"I'll try," she says, yawning. "If I can, I need to get my rest, right?" I see her pulling back her covers, and pulling them up to her neck as she curls up beneath them, smiling.

"You are definitely right," I agree. "Sleep well." She hangs up the phone, and I start getting ready for bed.

• • •

WELL. IT'S finally here! Graduation day! Two in the afternoon, here, and am I ever having difficulty with my black gown! Actually, it's not so much the gown as it is the hood. The hood is like a window curtain, only the dark blue satin fabric is supposed to drape around my shoulders, and the light blue stripes along the edges are supposed to bunch up at the back. It has to be folded properly. The

ELECTRIC

directions in the gown packet I purchased a while back make it look so easy. False advertising, in my opinion. My hood looks nothing like the picture.

What makes it worse, is the fact that I am running out of time. I am in line, waiting my turn to get my picture taken with my family at the Nittany Lion Shrine, the stone statue of Penn State's mascot. The people ahead of me are finishing up with their photo shoots relatively fast, and I am desperately asking anyone around me to help out. I can tell one or two families are getting agitated; some others are getting a kick out of my troubles. But no one seems to know how to fold the hood. After several failed attempts, I tell those people behind me to go on ahead. And after another series of faulty folding, my parents and grandparents agree that my back will be out of sight and we will worry about my appearance later.

The Lion Shrine is a beautiful sculpture, a gift given by a graduating class years ago, I think. It is one of the most visited tourist attractions on campus throughout the year, primarily during football season, but also on graduation day. Having a photo at this site on this triumphant day will bring back fond memories in the future, I'm sure.

I know that I will look back and recall the evenings I stopped walking along the brick sidewalk just to stand before the shining landmark, one hand on my hip, to admire the craftsmanship, to motivate myself to represent my university well, and to remind myself that God made me a Nittany Lion for a reason.

When all of my family have climbed and reached the peak of the mulch-strewn mound surrounding the shrine, we huddle close together as someone gladly takes our picture for us. To my right, my grandmother laughs hard, says, "Can you believe you've done it?" and makes sure my cap is on correctly, pushing my tassel aside so it isn't blocking my face. To my left, my grandpa is grinning, says, "What do ya' say, buddy? You ready?" and lovingly squeezes me. The camera flashes three times, and the lady taking the picture says, "Beautiful!"

After I have finished posing with Grandma and Grandpa, my father and I stand right next to the lion and hug each other. Grandpa takes several shots. It is extremely windy, my gown isn't deflecting it at all, and my hood is flailing, so Dad and I descend the mound, step around one of the lights that makes the famous cat glow at night, and walk to the car intent on going to the Performing Arts Building, where the graduation ceremony will take place.

I have to be there at three, and I should make it on time.

• • •

I ARRIVE AT the Performing Arts Building at three, exactly. My chest progressively pounds as I walk towards the entrance, my heartbeat increasing because I'm filled with emotion. I'm feeling eager, nervous, proud, and, I admit, even vulnerable. You name it; I'm feeling it. Climbing the stairs, I see other students in their gowns and caps, with their hoods improperly folded as well, and it eases my concerns about my attire.

Upon entering the building, I examine the layout of the foyer, the maroon carpeting, the soft maroon benches along the walls, and the table in the center, where I have to get my name tag with my

GRAND MAL

college and major printed on it. The doors to the auditorium are still closed, and, for the most part, except for a beautifully decorated conifer in the corner, the area is empty. The stillness and the beautiful décor makes me feel warm on the inside, slows my heartbeat some.

I walk up to the table lined in black, ruffled cloth and ask one of the three ushers in classy tuxedos to give me my name tag. The lady usher marks my name on the list, and kindly tells me not to lose the card because I'll have to hand it in before I go on stage. As I walk away from the table, I think, *Well, that was easy enough. Relax, Chris.* And my heartbeat becomes a slow patter.

Between observing the building and speaking with the ushers, I was so caught up in the moment, feeling so warm, that I didn't realize how many graduates and family members had come in. They are still coming through the front doors. Most of the graduates appear to be as emotional as I am, excited about graduating, but uncertain about ceremony protocol.

One thing they all are doing is repositioning gowns and hoods. Husbands are helping graduating wives. Wives are helping graduating husbands. Parents are helping their graduating sons and daughters. And Grandparents are helping graduating grandchildren.

I am intrigued by how differently people of other ethnic backgrounds are prepping themselves here. From what I've seen, the Asians are doing so in a reserved and thorough manner. The Africans seem to be the happiest, making small talk about the gowns. The African Americans are the most verbal, laughing loudly at their dressing difficulties. And the Whites appear to be satisfied with whatever works, somewhat indifferent about the whole thing.

JOSHUA HOLMES

My Grandparents and Parents are happily walking in my direction to help me prep. Only this time, an assistant who has helped graduates tidy up in the past is walking by their side to move the process forward more quickly, and, most importantly, make me look good. I have to say, that, after my tie is pulled tight, my gown is zipped up, my hood is in place, and my cap is on, I feel awesome.

Not long after the director has finished cleaning me up, and my family takes more pictures, do the other ushers open the doors to the auditorium, and point the graduates to separate doors, to find their colleges and stand in the assigned area until further notice. Before I do so, I glance back at my family, and see that everyone I invited, except for Michael and Linda, is here. Content, I go and find my college, The College of Education, by looking at the colors on the hood, and stand there with several students I have never seen or heard before.

I stand for a long time. I even talk to some of the students.

• • •

A FUNNY, OLDER gentleman in full, purple satin garb interrupts all the students in conversation. "We're starting soon, everyone. Let me look at your hoods!" He goes from person to person, turns the decorative pieces around when necessary, and gives us a history lesson on the origin of the dress. I hear him say "Way back in the day . . ." several times before we all line up.

Golden posts with vinyl ribbons are positioned so that I and my fellow graduates must march single file, as we all make our way into the auditorium, and descend the sloping walkway. The floor is

ELECTRIC

carpeted maroon, like in the foyer, and the walls are colored a light pink. Large cup- like, golden lights are evenly placed on an extended parapet, the place more formal than anything I've seen.

And the place is packed; let me tell you. I'm taken aback. Considering no one needed tickets to attend, I thought the place would almost be empty. Man was I wrong. Not only are the ground seats filled, but the seats in the balcony are, as well. I can't help but admire the carved, white concrete colonnades that support the balcony, too.

As I reach my reserved row of seats, I wait until the funny man instructs me to start towards my seat. I feel awkward walking in front of the already seated audience. This whole scene feels bigger than life. I accomplished a lot, yes, but all of this attention? I don't know. I'm a simple guy who doesn't like to receive a lot of public notice. "Holy Crap," I mutter. "This is crazy."

• • •

THE MAN who presents the commencement speech is a revered dean with numerous credentials President Graham Spanier, among others, finds valuable. The credentials mean nothing to me. He gives a crazy dialogue about climate change, the slow demise of human existence, and the graduates' role in making the general public aware of it. Apparently, he believes, we, "having achieved a level of education many have not," have a responsibility to go out into the world and promote change. A talk about climate change at a graduation ceremony? I don't know what the President was thinking!

After sitting almost forty-five minutes through the depressing dialogue, and thirty more minutes through the procession of the doctoral candidates, watching their professors hood their students, and the dean handing them their diplomas, the master's students in my row are instructed to stand and walk out of the auditorium, out to the area where I stood previously, to go to the back stairwell leading to the curtained platform, and, finally, to hand my name card into a woman who is responsible for telling me when to walk onstage.

As I wait, I think back to earlier in the day, the few moments just prior to my departure from the lobby, when I saw John conversing with Mrs. Patterson, no sign of animosity towards my professor, no indication in his face that his childhood was making it difficult to socialize with the lady I initially had difficulties with. She nodded her head repeatedly, smiled, and gazed at him deeply, her eyes full of empathy. Perhaps her sensitivity had helped him come to a realization that he could overcome his past.

And, right behind John and Mrs. Patterson, I saw Sam and Alex laughing with one another; the old man patting my friend on the back, encouraging him, I'm sure. Alex's forehead was plastered in creases, fissures of happiness, to my delight. Sam had his dreads neatly pulled back into a ponytail of sorts, his minimal attempt at formality. I felt good seeing two people so different so satisfied with each other's company at an event honoring my achievement.

Back in the present, I hear a "psssst." I look behind me, at the woman who I handed my name card to. "It's your turn. Start walking." This is the moment I've been waiting for, for two long years. I take a deep breath, soak up the moment, and commit it to memory. In my long gown, I glide onto the stage and do as the Doctoral students did, shake hands with the president, and the deans. Over the

GRAND MAL

speakers, I hear my name and major called out. *Finally!* I think. *It is over!* I look out into the crowd, watching for my family and friends.

I spot them all half way across the platform. Talk about an absolute, a truth no one can dispute. Not Plato. Not Aristotle. Not anyone! When I see my Parents and Grandparents, Sam, John, Alex, and my angel Mary Grace, the view is as vivid as any I would see in a dream during a seizure. Only this is not a dream. And I am definitely not having a Grand Mal.

THE END

SEIZURE
A NOVELLA

AUTHOR OF GRAND MAL
JOSHUA HOLMES

PART ONE

PROLOGUE
IN THE CAR

I FELL BACK towards him even though he kept pushing my body away. Over and over I tilted left, towards the cup holder, the driver's side, only to reverse tilt a second later, precipitating more shoves. I shook until my body was a dead weight again, motor skills gone for now, but I fought it. And so did he. One hand on the steering wheel, the other, to an extent, hoisting my body up, he was afraid and I was afraid.

I'd normally respond positively to the mechanics of a buckle, but the resistance of the seatbelt against my chest and at my waist frightened me. I began to panic. There was this delayed unconscious moment I've yet to figure out when my brain recognized I was scared, and it somehow sent me into an even deeper state of adrenaline-laced terror.

I frantically tugged at the seatbelt. Pulled hard. Yanked with all my might, no sense at all in my actions. I continued to yank, toiling obsessively without rationale.

I profusely apologized to him, sorry that he had to witness this mess that was me. I did this every time. Was my action driven by guilt?

"It's OK, Chris," he said. "I'm here."

My throat burned. It was raw from trying to fill my lungs, to catch my breath. My chest was full of phlegm. I coughed.

The car was still moving, on the highway. High beams coming from the opposite direction nearly blinded him, nearly blinded me. I could hear myself crying, panting, could vaguely see my reflection in the passenger window.

"Chris. You had a seizure."

I let out a cry. The black macadam raced towards us, and it felt the yellow double lines would come right through the windshield.

"I can't breathe."

"I know. I am going to pull over, okay?"

"I'm so hot."

Hand to my forehead, I pushed my brown hair aside, dabbed sweat from beneath my bangs, and wiped it on my jeans. I was exhausted.

I saw cars pass us. Some drivers laid on the horn. Others shook their heads in disgust. And others still offered nasty hand gestures.

"You want the fans toward you? Just let me pull over."

SEIZURE

He turned the car off a nearby exit, and pulled into a gas station. We just sat there, together, and tried to gather ourselves as best we could, considering.

He turned the fans on the dashboard in my direction.

"I can't take this anymore," I said, leaning forward. In that moment, I honestly didn't think I could.

• • •

1
JUST ANOTHER PLACE

AT ANOTHER place, but in the same position, I deduced; a different time, I sensed, but in the same splayed trajectory. Like a man on the cross, my left hand lay near my head to be anchored. And on the opposite side, my right hand waited as well. On my back, even my legs were overlapped, and I frantically looked up and then side-to-side, trying to figure it all out. Lots of people. Frowning faces. Heads shaking. Whispering. Worrying. I had to be in public. Subway? Starbucks? Each location very possible.

Green. All around its green. Pine counters. Pine tables. Pine floor mats. Employees in pine aprons. No yellow in the sign above me, just a female in a pine crown and pine stripes. Enough for me to decide I was at Starbucks.

A bulky lady hovered over me. "I am an EMT in Baltimore," she said. "He needs to stay still until the ambulance gets here."

JOSHUA HOLMES

I had to stay still? Not again. With a deep breath, I tried to hoist myself up onto my elbows, to look around and soak up more of my surroundings but exhaustion overcame me.

The bulky lady pointed at a woman with several whiny young children. "Please take your kids outside, ma'am."

Geesh, I thought. *Do they really have to make such a big deal out of me? Am I that scary?* I couldn't remember everything I did or didn't, whether or not I shook, but I found it hard to believe it warranted all this attention.

Stone, the manager, stood in his pine apron a few feet away, leaning on a broom stick, and asked, "Are you all right, Chris?"

"I'm ok. I had a seizure."

The bulky lady interrupted. "You sure did, honey. Lay down. You hit your head pretty hard, too."

I HAD HIT my head. That's what Bulky said anyway. For the life of me, though, I couldn't find a knot or a tender spot. I rubbed my skull as I thought about things and waited for the ambulance.

I looked at the floor to locate a point of impact. I thought perhaps I had left a visible mark, but I didn't see blood or a burnished tile.

I saw my black, leather computer bag a short distance away. My computer was in there. All my ideas. My contact information for my current clients. What I once used for graduate work in the counseling field, I now used to assist me with freelance graphic design. I couldn't lose my computer or anything on it, otherwise I could kiss next month's paycheck goodbye. When you are pinned on your back, however, it's hard to collect any belongings.

ELECTRIC

I was disappointed to see the fabric had been ripped, I assumed, from the fall. The outside netting that held my pens and pencils was torn from corner to corner. Beyond the tear, though, the bag seemed alright.

The bag reminded me why I had visited Starbucks that day. It wasn't even a week prior when a pastor had contacted me about designing the interior and exterior of a children's book. We agreed to meet at the coffee shop to discuss all the technicalities and the cost. I now recalled it had gone as planned and I had reached an agreement with him.

I was having a decent day, went on to call and tell a friend about my good fortune. In that moment, however, I started losing my speech, the dreaded pre-cursor. I tried to talk my way through it, heard my friend asking if I was okay, but the next thing I knew, I couldn't speak at all. I dropped my phone, turned sideways, and twisted hard to the right until I tipped back in my chair.

IT ALL could have ended as formulaically as most commercial movies do today, my story I mean, but then again, where's the reality in that? My story continues. I imagine if you are reading this, I didn't traumatize you enough the first time around, and you are back for more. Well don't fret, there's plenty to tell you. Honestly, friends, as far as my Epilepsy is concerned, I still have it and the condition still manifests itself in ways beyond the average person's active imagination.

I didn't change my name, Chris, either, since I've yet to hear that any such change would affect the attributes of my Epilepsy. I know it's not a name with a lot of gusto, but it will grow on you. As far as I know, I could be a Frank, Charlie, or Mo, and still have to endure the thrills of my diagnosis.

I hope you catch my dry tone when I speak of "thrills." It's anything but thrilling. Several years after my fall from a seizure into the ditch in State College, PA, however, I am again preparing myself for a wild night of "thrills." All I can do is be a little sarcastic about it.

In any case, today really did start like most others. Sorry if that sounds cliché. And I should clarify that it started like any other day after my graduation from PSU and design school, and following my decision to pursue an art and design profession.

It was the beginning of December, a nice holiday reminder although the rest of the world seemed to have started celebrating in October. My room was a little chillier than normal, but it felt nice to cuddle a bit longer before convincing myself to rise and dress.

I noticed my torso and neck ached as I put my shirt on, and the comforters on my bed were askew, indicators of a seizure-filled night I couldn't recall. After I finally gathered my things, I decided to head out into the world. I didn't foresee an ambulance visit.

CHRIS. CAN you walk?" Another big-boned woman asked, the local EMT I guessed.

I was shaky, no question. Shaky and weak. I rubbed my knees, and took another deep breath. I felt the cold, textured tiles underneath me. "I should be able to."

I looked for the woman's name tag. I was disoriented, but finally located it, there with her title. She offered me a hand and said, "My name's Sally."

SEIZURE

"And I'm June." The second EMT, rosy in the cheeks and slightly beefier, offered me a hand too.

I thought I vaguely recognized them both from a previous occurrence at another venue. I hoped for this so that I might convince them to consider what had happened in my other instance, and, bottom line, to forget protocols that just didn't work.

All the green around me disappeared, the decorative air vents and overbearing, duo-tone wall mural, as I was pushed unbuckled out the door into the bitter cold and falling white snow.

June said, "I do remember you." And then she went on to take down personal information from my silver, medic alert bracelet, among other things.

Once strapped into the aluminum gurney, the two local EMTs lifted me into the back of the ambulance with relative ease. From my perch, I stared out the vehicle's rear at the snowdrift and waited.

For those who've never been in this position, I can only describe it as surreal. A person can only be objectified so much until he or she goes into a self-protective mode. I went there whenever I was forced to lay within these tight confines.

But I eventually had to answer all the questions on their medical forms, and they called the ER, even though I would have preferred to sign release of service forms and head home.

More bluntly, I would've preferred the old way— when I had a say in my medical affairs. Now they performed the medical "services" first—the electro-cardiogram, the blood sugar test, the blood pressure test, to name a few—and then put my rights in the hands of the doctor on call, only reminding me of the charges after the fact, if prompted.

I understood that the EMTs had to make a living, don't get me wrong, but the hospital visit was pointless, like most of them. Yet it was beyond my control.

You see, what happens is this: by the time I arrive at the Emergency Room, my body has recovered, which ties everyone's hands. That particular night, I was wheeled out into the bright, ER hallway, left to wait. I didn't even have an assigned room. I enlightened the doctors though. "My body hurts all over," I said to half a dozen different physicians. "But I'll survive. No tests please."

• • •

2
THE CALL

I DIDN'T KNOW how to respond the day I received the call. It was random and brought up a lot of emotions I didn't even realize were still there. I knew I had attempted to block things out, to push it down for self-preservation, but I guess the hurt had just been covered by something else and left to sit deep inside.

That particular phone ring startled me, too, because I had been intently focused on assembling one of my design projects. I think I had been simultaneously watching a YouTube tutorial on unique font combinations, Photoshop filters, or something like that, and a TV talk show, when I was jarred back to reality.

"It's me, Chris. Michael." My former best friend.

I muted the TV, was silent a minute, then said, "I know, Michael. Hi."

ELECTRIC

I hadn't talked to Michael, or his new wife, Linda, since the day they officially quit school, since they left my apartment, a semester prior to my graduation in Penn State.

They both chose not to attend my ceremony, and I hadn't been invited to their wedding. I mean, I did tell Michael I thought he was stupid for dropping out, regardless of whether or not he was in love, which didn't go over real well, but I wouldn't have been a good friend if I silently agreed with every emotional thought he had and didn't give him some logic to mull over.

And that cross tattoo he had inked onto his wrist? Such a permanent mark! I never gave him grief over it, but to this day, I shook my head at the thought. Perhaps a popular move back then, I wondered if he'd regret it later.

In any case, while I accepted his decisions, I didn't like how things happened, and how we all had moved on without addressing the divide that inevitably emerged.

While I knew Michael and Linda were philosophy lovers, I couldn't tell you if either of them used the area of study professionally. And I didn't know if they debated for leisure any longer. I hadn't inquired about job choices, their general life direction, or anything else for that matter, and I still ached in my gut too much to ask or say anything that surpassed surface chatter.

I turned off the TV, shut down my computer, disconnected it from my surge protector, and set it aside.

"I'm coming to York later this week, Chris," said Michael. "Thought I'd call you up. It's been a while."

JOSHUA HOLMES

I turned over onto my back, spread eagle on the mattress, taking in the news.

A while? To put it mildly, I thought. He hadn't talked to me in ages!

"It has been a while."

IT AMAZED me what came to mind on my back after I set the phone down. The color of Michael's hair: red if he hadn't changed it. His quip, "Back to the good life." Whether he still said it constantly as he rubbed his goatee. Whether he still cooked awesome-smelling pancakes and nasty-smelling curry, or if he changed these habits to appease Linda. Women do mold their men, after all.

My mind jumped to our childhood. How long we had been friends. Our afternoons in the back yard. Our innocent talks about everyday discoveries.

It then jumped to his scar—my scar too—and our brain surgeries. His success, my botched procedure. His seizure-free life, my seizure-filled life. But I moved on quickly.

I jumped to Penn State, to college; remembered how close we were, and how separated we became. How his relationship with Linda ruined everything. Made Michael dismiss logic and fear my condition like everyone else under the sun. How it ultimately made me stronger, but less inclined to socialize.

I WAS WAITING for the bus again, thinking about my response to Michael's call, how I could be a good host, if I should be one in the first place. Shuffling my cold feet on the narrow berm of Queen Street, just beyond Waters Road, I could vaguely see over the mounds of salted snow the back of the older house into which I

SEIZURE

had recently moved. The relatively small, surrounding community, the bright neon lights of Suburban Bowlerama, Enterprise Rent-a-car, the powder blue exterior of the next door TV station, Fox 43, and a lot of speeding cars, as well.

The Red Rabbit bus was late again, because it was almost impossible to keep a schedule with holiday traffic, I knew. It would normally bother me, but I was busy thinking about my options as it pertained to Michael's visit. I didn't doubt my ability to act as a disconnected tour guide. It was the required, one-on-one interaction that at one point came so easily to me.

If it were anyone else, I wouldn't think twice about the meeting. Bottom line, I know myself well enough to see that I was allowing my emotions to rule, and I needed to get over my hang-ups quickly if I was to offer any semblance of decency.

I'd heard so many pastors and motivational speakers talk about the immediate choice to remain imprisoned, or to move on after a life hurdle, and how the choice affected the future; Though perplexed by the teaching at times, I didn't doubt that it was true. In fact, just then, I thought that the philosophy would be applicable here, and would resolve my dilemma if I could only speedily put it into action.

I chuckled to myself because I realized I had considered an unlikely possibility: speedy decision-making. Never would I, Chris, be speedy. Ever. It was just not a part of me. Fortunately, no one saw my random snicker, and I stroked my goatee to hide my smile and manage my expression.

I then adjusted my computer bag on my shoulder, and leaned on my dominant leg. I sighed and looked eagerly up the road for the red bus. Michael and I had been long-time friends. How could I just let that go? It would temporarily ease my angst, but not for long. I would eventually feel guilty.

I grasped my red bus pass tightly, and stuffed my hand into my deep coat pocket. A half hour later, the heavy whoosh of bus breaks sounded. As I stepped into the bus and swiped my card, I decided to pray about my situation and do the logical thing: stop dwelling on what was, and take everything one day at a time. *Re-focus and push on*, I thought.

• • •

3
LOOKING BACK

ANYONE WHO knew me well would confirm that I did my best work when I was troubled. Not such an unusual claim since many artists and designers throughout history composed moody masterpieces via creativity and free expression during tumultuous times.

While the feelings of tumult that inspired me were personal, and only emerged on occasion, in my opinion, I used them productively to complete portrait and animal drawings in pastel, colored pencil, and digital software, and did so to earn some extra money.

Over the years I had accrued quite a collection that affirmed my talent, encouraged clients to seek my specific style, and made school a lot easier to complete, as I had images around which to conceptualize.

ELECTRIC

Upon acquiring an illustration job, I usually set garbage bags or old towels on the floor area near my small closet. From that closet, I pulled out my blue duffel bag and orange suitcase chock full of supplies I've also accumulated over the years, a piece of suede mat board, and set to work in the inspired zone.

This was a practice that went back to my late high school days. I spent hours in the dank basement, by myself in the empty space. Under the grey lighting, I pondered over a piece, next to my stockpile of supplies, talk radio in the background.

Between my personal and professional life concerns, my spike in public seizure frequency, and my former friend's upcoming visit, I had plenty of inspiration to rely upon.

I had drawn for such a long time that, unlike many artists who drew out of fear, I composed with confidence. I recognized that inspired place, and created when it was there. I didn't worry about achieving a likeness of my subject, because I knew I'd eventually get there, regardless of any flaws in the process. As an artist, all I had to capture was a likeness. The degree of desired realism was relative, depending on who looked at the reference, and, ultimately, on who paid.

It took years, but after completing design school, I reached a point where I trusted my own judgment. I hadn't done anything, artistically speaking, that warranted a spirit of self-distrust, and in my mind, that was a major accomplishment.

LOOKING BACK, I accomplished a lot this year. I mean I try my best to succeed every year in everything I do; and to overcome my failures with other accomplishments. But this year, specifically, was a productive one.

JOSHUA HOLMES

Not everyone can say they graduated from Penn State followed by design school with honors and worked independently in the same field of study. I understand, however, the difference between doing several temporary projects, and building a client base for future projects and sustained business growth. My aim this year was to endure.

Like anything else, independent work had its challenges, the unpredictability for instance, but, so far, it seemed freelance design also had its perks: it suited my personality and presented an obtainable opportunity as far as making a living was concerned. I tried to keep it all in perspective, that life happened in stages, and experiences and opportunities came in waves, either temporarily knocking me down or surprising me with a new avenue to pursue. Sometimes I accepted it; other times, I struggled to. In any case, I can't endure too many of these platitudes, but can say that I'm interested to see what happens this upcoming year.

When there were opportunity droughts this past year, I took it upon myself to expand my knowledge base. It didn't take long—well, several interview rejections over a period of months, actually—to see that employers wanted graphic designers with web literacy. I took business and online courses in web coding and development: HTML, CSS, PHP, and JavaScript. While I did grasp the languages and design a website, I had more success in image manipulation, logo design, and corporate identity, and even more success in my lifelong specialty, illustration.

SEIZURE

In my view, it just goes to show that we as humans are meant to find our talents, the gifts about which we are passionate, and pursue them either personally or professionally.

THE PASTOR seemed to agree with me the day we met at Starbucks. I shared my sentiments about using personal gifts, a little of my life story to break the ice, and he thanked me for being so open. He told me of the small church he led, of the pride he felt for the growing congregation, of the direction he wanted to see the church go, and made some general inquiries about my spiritual state and church attendance before moving onto our project.

"So tell me about your idea," I prompted that day. "Where I come into play . . ."

The pastor was a thin man; not Fed-Ex guy skinny, but not wrestler-heavy either. He smiled constantly as he sipped on his coffee. Took his time, too.

"Well, Chris." Slow sip. "I need an illustrator."

My ears perked up at the sound of a job. It was my area of expertise. I bit into a chocolate chip cookie, thought, *Amen brother!*

"And what do you need illustrated?" I asked, more personally than a car salesman, but less than a shrink. "It's a special ministry opportunity, actually Chris."

He went on to slowly describe his idea, to tell me of a story he wanted to develop, not unlike many that other of my clients had before.

"A ministry for kids," he added.

I briefly brought out a drawing pad and my laptop, and showed my skills. "I can illustrate something for kids on paper first, then use the Adobe Suite, and design anything else you might need."

"I know you can." His smile broadened. I sensed he was confident in me, and it did feel good.

"Any typographic preferences?" I probed. "Font families that you like?"

"Just pick something fun." I nodded and told him I could do that too. We talked about my fee, and shook on it minutes later.

I was excited because I had used some of my counseling skills, built rapport with a potential long-term client, and done so on my terms.

I intended to lie on my bed as long as necessary, to conceptualize, and design in front of my Mac for many, many hours to help fulfill the pastor's dream and earn my compensation.

• • •

4
NEVER FORGOT HER

MARY GRACE'S presence was one that I never forgot, or even tried to for that matter. And I think the reason was two-fold: 1) she had always been the girl who made me feel special whether in grade school, high school, in college, or afterward, and 2) as a nurse at my current neurology clinic, she epitomized everything wonderful the rest of the nurse triage wasn't to me.

She made the appointments bearable. We both knew each visit would go the same way, bogged down by doctoral egotism, intru-

ELECTRIC

sive government procedures, and ultimately impacted by the most recent Epilepsy drug recommendations, which I always declined.

We both would later laugh about all the ludicrous side effects that came with the recommendations, how the doctors listed them matter-of-factly, commercial-like, and then justified them by saying, "The company says it only happens to two percent." As if I'd never been that two percent before. And then how the staff looked in my direction, waiting for me to say, "Sure thing doc, can't wait for the blue fingernails, double vision, possible blindness, and, if I'm lucky, constant weariness."

Mary Grace always looked at me kindly from behind the doctor, with genuine empathy like she used to in the grade school gym, or high school football stands when I was upset I couldn't participate in sports, and her eyes just said, "Let it go." And I usually could.

I was beyond that idyllic association I once had, the notion that she was angelic and had a halo in my mind's eye, but I wasn't above saying that she was different, that she was in a class of her own, and that she left a lasting impression.

Since she gave me a nice check up, accepted my graduation ceremony invite, and attended the event, I had thought a lot about her, whether she had hidden baggage, whether she dated, whether she had kids, whether she thought about me.

I also said to myself, "Well, Chris, you invited her once ... why not do it again?" And I debated the question, always debating in my head.

One day, I'd work up the nerve.

• • •

5
CONCENTRATION

Until then, I had to concentrate on finding interested clients similar to the pastor. That's to say, clients with authenticity, with a confidence and strong sense of trust in me, perhaps clients with an urgency to achieve their dreams.

While the aforementioned customer type was ideal, at the end of the day, I was open to finding any client. I knew they wouldn't all be like the pastor, which made each opportunity unique.

There were so many design opportunities out there, but twice, if not triple, the number of designers. And there was always someone better. I had to set myself apart, apply the standard marketing strategy of service/ product positioning. I had to find that one angle that nobody had yet approached.

I was different in that I had knowledge in other areas of study, English and Counseling, but in our current economy this fact seemed more of a detriment than anything, seemed to make employers think twice, to question why I hadn't gone further.

One thing I observed in school, though, was that students were either good or bad writers. Students were both fluid and poetic with their concepts and taglines, or they just missed the mark entirely. I happened to excel in the English area, and I made it a goal to offer editing and manuscript compilation services in addition to book cover design whenever I could. It wasn't necessarily unique to me, but it was a necessity for those who wanted to preserve the standards of traditional publishing, and no one in my immediate network followed suit.

I had considered taking it a step further, investing in my own website, postcards, newspaper and online banner ads. My electronic portfolio was substantial and had received plenty of notice, but it, too, could use an update.

I wasn't naïve, however. I was aware that, regardless of my positioning, of my ads, I had to re-visit my interview approach. It was complicated, I knew—so many factors at play—but a wrinkle that in time God would iron out.

• • •

6
EXTRA MEASURES

EVERY NOW and again, when there was a lull in freelance work, I would contact my design school to see if they had any job leads. I had started visiting the Career Services office weeks before graduation to test the touted hundred percent job placement rating, and I never let up until I started pulling in my own clients with regularity.

I worked with a woman named Terrence Pincher. She was a spunky, trim, dark-haired lady in her fifties, I guessed, and her approachable air was perfect for the role. Her demeanor was engaging, and her raspy voice and throaty intonation was infectious.

I had called her a lot, initially. Probably more than I could recall. The early bird caught the worm, right? Why my peers never seemed to grasp this concept always amazed me, but their inactivity really did work to my advantage. And I wasn't surprised when she bellowed a loud, "Why hello there, Chris! What can I do for you?"

"Hi Terrence. How are you? Just calling to see if you had any freelance work for me."

"Doing well, here." A pause. "Actually Chris, I think I do."

"Awesome. Thanks so much."

"Let me see here. I have a name and number around somewhere." She let out a laugh as she rustled through her files.

I asked her what was going on at the school, if the annual portfolio show had gone well. Her answer usually told me whether or not it was a good time to call.

Aside from the graduation ceremony, the show was the pinnacle moment of the semester for Terrence, which required a lot of her time and energy.

"Oh the show went splendidly . . . a good turn out. And things are settling down now, so I have a few minutes to chat."

"Well I have a pen here, whenever you are ready." Terrence had several other graduates for whose employment status she was responsible, so I was glad to get her attention.

She gave me a number to a potential employer, explained that he wanted to grow his start-up and expressed interest in someone like me. I wrote it all down, excited for the opportunity.

• • •

ELECTRIC

7
PREPARATION

IT OCCURRED to me that I had two options for Michael as it related to sleeping at my place, and the second option was definitely more optimal for us both. He could either 1.) take my bed, while I took the couch—which tended to be uncomfortable—or 2.) I could stay in my own bed and room, and pick up a cheap inflatable mattress and charger at Bon Ton for my former best friend.

I didn't see the need to present the options, as I really wanted to sleep in my own bed, and I imagined Michael would prefer his own sleeping station.

There were places, I knew, that rented the noted items, but I was leery of that sort of thing, as I associated a rental with last resorts, and I wouldn't own the items for future use.

A Queensgate Plaza regular, I stopped by the strip mall Bon Ton on a mission shortly after, and thoroughly searched the premises for a reasonable, blow-up bed and battery charger. While the store never had applied a solid marketing and sales strategy, I occasionally found a deal hidden underneath the misleading signage.

I searched carefully, more quickly than I would elsewhere too, as the store was plastered in fluorescent lights, which often triggered seizures. I was sensitive to the brightness, and always had been.

I recalled when, back in the day, the chain had been one of the upscale types, and how it had later changed. Over the years, this particular store turned into an unusual hybrid of low-end and renowned products and clotheslines catered to the local neighborhoods. It primarily relied on overstock sales and coupons, and yet it remained open and relatively busy.

I often wondered how much longer it would survive. So many other stores had either closed their doors or gone bankrupt under the current administration.

In any case, I hated to part with eighty bucks, fifty for the mattress, thirty for the charger, but it was a need, and I would be able to use them more than once.

Upon arriving home, I unfolded the bed and uncapped the plug, tested the charger, loud and slow though it was, and a couple hours later, pushed the mattress against the wall at the end of my own bed.

Sleeping arrangements were settled. I now had one less thing to be concerned about.

PEOPLE DIDN'T seem to understand that, following a seizure in a public place, the person with Epilepsy had to ponder at home what happened, over and over, and muster the courage to go back to the place where they felt powerless and a sense of shame.

And to complicate matters, while he or she knew that the situation required attention, it was unwanted, and would most likely precipitate a change in how people treated them.

I didn't make this up. Even the ER nurse had given me a packet on the subject—which must have some merit—before I gladly departed my hospital cell. For whatever reason, I kept the packet up on my bureau.

SEIZURE

Nevertheless, I wrestled with the issue while wrestling with the inflatable mattress that, until I later mastered the process, was more of a deflatable mattress than anything.

As I finished up with the inflatable bed, I had an urge for coffee. But that involved me heading back into the world. Sounded rational, right? Except I relived the seizure repeatedly in my head, and if I had to go face Stone, the Starbucks manager again, or endure another incident, I was sure I would scream. I even considered just staying in.

I also knew, however, that staying in meant I was living life fearfully. And I wasn't about to adjust for fear. I had done it too often in the past, and I was stronger now.

People asked me if my embarrassment was a matter of misperception. I despised that word so much. It was a politician's term. A relativist's term. In this context, though, perhaps it was a relevant point. And yet individual perception, in my view, was a person's reality, my reality.

• • •

8
FEARS CONFIRMED

STONE DID in fact confirm my fears. He treated me with a forced kindness I recognized from others who witnessed my seizures. When I re-entered Starbucks, again leaning on a broom in a green apron, he shouted, "Hey there, buddy! What can I get for you today?" Everybody turned and looked in my direction. I wanted to cower. The greeting wasn't that extreme, but it was different enough that it felt insincere and unnatural.

He could have been nasty or totally ignored me, and that would have felt worse, so I had to give him that much. Plenty of people had given me the cold shoulder after a seizure. I know everybody copes differently, but often it forced me to affirm people that I was fine, when, in actuality, I was in recovery.

Even now, it was hard to believe I was on the floor under the air vents and duo-tone mural a week prior. On the cold floor, shaking in the dirt. I had difficulty accepting it.

And there was no way that thought wasn't running through Stone's mind, as well. Even the best of feigners would fail to convince me otherwise.

"I'd like a Java chip Frappuccino," I said. "A venti, please." Stone, who was never previously an emphatic person, nodded his shiny, bald head with an exuberance that just didn't fit the request. I thought, *Way to overcompensate, there, Stone.*

"We have a special, today, buddy. A buy one, get one free, if you are interested."

I wasn't about to pass up a special, even if I got it on account of my disability. My take on it was this: if people felt better about the situation by gifting me with specials, I wasn't going to turn them down. I'm sensitive like that.

"Sure," I said. "Thank you. Sounds good."

• • •

ELECTRIC

9
EMERGENCE

STRANGE AS it might sound, the knot that I was certain would emerge on my head in fact never did. Delayed though it was, however, a week after my seizure, a piercing muscle spasm overcame my right shoulder, and proceeded to shoot bullets of pain into my mid-to-lower back and the base of my skull.

At first, I didn't consider it anything beyond another severe injury. But, as the days passed, I worried I might get addicted to the phone-prescribed pain pills. The spasms dulled with heavy muscle relaxants only to flare up again. I started to grow restless. The stabs were distracting and wouldn't stop nagging me.

Because I had sensory issues in my right side, the jolts were hard to settle and difficult to explain. I imagined they were akin to a wounded soldier's phantom pains and remember later contradicting myself when I said, "It's like a dull ache with sharp jabs."

As I went about my business, though, I noticed it was affecting my mood, and, in general, I just didn't want to be around anyone. I hurt too badly. Yet I knew I had to do something to alleviate the severity of my acquired injury.

So I attempted to consult with my neurologist, only to be put on hold when the nurse triage was preoccupied, and later referred to my primary doctor for reasons I've yet to find out.

After struggling to get solid answers from the specialists, I made an appointment with my primary doctor, and I crossed my fingers that I would leave the office with a legitimate treatment plan or credible diagnosis (although my Grandmother already diagnosed me with a concussion, as she had accurately done so often before).

• • •

10
HELPING

IN THE past, I'd been counseled to help others to keep perspective, told that it would solve my personal plagues. I tried it, and it didn't. Once I assisted at the YMCA. Another time I helped the church feed the poor. Did it take my mind off myself? Temporarily, yes. And did I feel a joy in helping others? Sure. Until, against my will, I was a public spectacle. And it happened more often than not.

I wanted with all my heart for the mere act of helping someone else to place all focus elsewhere. I wanted a random moment assisting an elderly person enter a church to resolve my pain problem.

Keeping focus was always a noble pursuit. At one time, I'd also been advised not to get distracted, that it was important to keep my eye on the prize.

At the same time, I knew the very fact that I wanted to help in order to overcome a crippling ache was a selfish desire, and couldn't be justified.

That was the catch-22 with the pain attack. So often, I had heard the clichés about mind over matter, how I could decide whether or not it would dictate the course of my life. It called to mind some of these extreme reality shows that demanded unrealistic living standards in the worst possible conditions.

I seemed to be losing the battle.

• • •

11
TECHNOLOGY BENEFITS

I NEVER THOUGHT I'd be one of these smart phone guys. But, as a confessed convert, I admit that once you leave dumb phones behind, there's no going back. Long time Apple fanatic though I might be, I hadn't expected to enjoy the upgraded cell's ease of use to the extent that I have.

And, believe it or not, it had nothing to do with the TV ads playing the latest pop hit in the background, exhibiting a one-word tagline noting the simplicity of the latest and greatest features.

For me, it was the visual experience: the colorful display, the streamlined apps, the organization that it provided. When the green voicemail app boasted a message it always excited me; made me wonder who wanted to speak with me.

Upon hearing the message, an inquiry from Mary Grace on behalf of the neurology clinic, I thought of her sitting there in a hallway chair, by the phone on the wall, the cord bouncing as she tugged the receiver, file cabinets and scale not far away. I was surprised to an extent: surprised by the immediacy of the call, but not surprised that it was my favorite nurse making the call.

"Hello Chris," she said over the phone. "I was sorry to hear you hurt yourself. Calling to check on the status of your head and neck injuries. Do me a favor and call the office. Ask for me."

I couldn't help but smile to myself. She cared enough to check on me. My expression would have been different, sour probably, if the other triage nurses had called.

I knew Mary Grace was doing her job; that she was following up. But I couldn't recall the last time a doctor or nurse reached out to me. I was always the one making contact attempts.

Mary Grace never ceased to amaze me.

• • •

12
REVELATION

AFTER THE Late Night Show with Jay Leno, one of his final monologues, I turned off the TV, pulled my covers to my chin, and closed my eyes to clear my head and pray. I talked to God for awhile. Afterward, I assessed what I had accomplished since mid-2013, a mental inventory if you will. What could I do to improve my situation? I wondered in the dark.

I was recalling what made me feel a sense of pride, what made me want to achieve a higher level of something, what made me invigorated.

Not to get super introspective or anything, but my mind wandered. I'm human. I thought about how I had spent so many years trying to please people; how it led to so much internal strain and emotional pain.

I even considered whether or not it was wise or healthy to go down that route, to think about such things since God pre-determined my path; whether or not I was exposing my mind to unnecessary stress.

Needless to say, my mind wouldn't stop.

I thought about my years studying karate, the few months Michael put in with me, the physical and mental challenge, performance-based and independent of opinion. Not my school studies. Not my design work. Karate.

It then occurred to me that, when studying karate, I also had pain issues, but the pursuit of physical and mental strength offset the battle wounds. It was pain with a purpose.

Here I was, in a latter life stage, trying to re-focus because the seizures and everything they entailed clouded my view, and it again hit me: I needed pain with a purpose.

• • •

13
PROCESSING

I DIDN'T THINK much more about Michael's random call in the next couple days or the blow-up mattress at the end of my bed because, before I knew it, his arrival time had come. I expected he would let me know when he made it to York. Until then, I'd make sure my place was suitable for a visit and try not to trip over the battery charger.

For so many years I watched my parents invest all their time and energy into hosting preparations for visiting family and friends, into carpet cleaning, bed making, into dinner planning, and so on. Admirable as it was, I wasn't about to put a bunch of money out for Michael. I would provide him with the essentials. Perhaps I would feel more generous in the future.

I did have an extra set of blankets and sheets, and a spare pillow and pillowcase that I pulled from my small closet and placed at the end of the blow-up. It escaped me earlier, but it hit me before it was too late.

Each day, as I prepared, I processed Michael's call and our shared past, and it grew a little easier to accept. I didn't feel the weight that initially pressured me, the conflict that occupied my mind.

We hadn't talked about anything substantial on the phone. I wished I hadn't been so caught off guard. We could have closed our past and paved the way for his visit to come.

But I failed to ask what he might want to do while in York. I hadn't prompted him about the matter, and he hadn't offered any indications. Perhaps we could catch a bite or attend a movie. Time would tell.

The weather was definitely inclement. But having walked the campus terrain for so many years, and now the uneven, wooded hillside along the roads, I was used to it. And I imagined Michael would be too, since he had to walk Linda home in similar State College conditions, and now whenever they went out together. It shouldn't pose a barrier, but worst-case scenario, we'd stay inside.

• • •

14
STORMS

I HAD ALWAYS loved the sound of storms: the sprinkle and pounding of rain, the static in the air, and the sporadic claps of thunder that followed fissures of lightning.

I loved listening to the wind whip the tree branches just outside my bedroom windows over and over against the wooden panes, to the house creak under the force.

I loved how, psychologically speaking, the stormy sounds of York made me feel a sense of peace and safety. I'm not sure where that feeling originated, but it might explain why, for years, I fell asleep to a sound machine with dripping water as its primary noise cycle.

But when I couldn't make time for said sounds, similar noises that immersed the bowling alley were the next best things. I thought about this the day I walked over to Suburban Bowlerama to inquire about a league.

I was not optimistic about leagues because it was early in the year, and they always seemed to cost an arm and leg, but I was pleasantly surprised. I saw the familiar face of Marge, the owner's wife, behind the counter, and I decided to ask about any available programs.

I had noticed, coming in, that a program for retirees was in progress. The older participants didn't seem to have a care in the world. I so wanted to experience that degree of nonchalance, and hoped for good news, for a program geared to younger people.

"As a matter of fact, honey, we have one starting next week."

"Wonderful," I said, leaning forward. "Do you have any info I can take with me?"

"Right here, honey." She handed me a flyer with a signup form attached.

I filled out the details, detached them for Marge, thanked her as she took the form, and headed home.

WHEN I got home, I unfolded the flyer to check out the specifics of the league. It was a "Pizza, Beer, & Bowl" league that took place every Wednesday night at 9:15 PM. It didn't require any previous experience, was relatively cheap if you paid weekly or monthly, and it just seemed downright fun. I wouldn't have any alcohol, but I expected to eat a few pizza slices and down a few sodas in between strike attempts. I planned to get my money's worth.

I admit that I had no clue what I was getting into. For all I knew, I could walk into the sequel of *The Big Lebowski*, whatever that meant. Beyond a former roommate's claim that the movie was a bowling classic, I only knew it consisted of an impressive cast but, otherwise, was unfamiliar with the plot, so my experience could also be something entirely different.

As far as building a social life was concerned, however, it could only improve via the league. Aside from going out with a few longtime friends every so often, I had grown sedate, and this new membership opportunity was something that I looked forward to.

• • •

PART TWO

15
WAVELENGTHS

MURKY AND dark, my room was painted navy and adorned with long, floor-to-ceiling curtains that pushed away the falling snow's white hue, except for a narrow strip at the window's edge. I rubbed my achy neck as I pulled the curtains closer together. In that moment, it seemed the pain would never end.

Different wavelengths mess with my brain and my stubborn curtains were just then as well. I closed my eyes in a weak attempt to negate the pain and escape the two competing wavelengths, the darkness, the strip of light. I then opened my eyes when I realized I was just welcoming further spasms and light-induced nightmares.

"Please God," I said. "Spare me, please." For the millionth time, it felt, I was met with a silent, hollow noise.

I buttoned my pants in front of the window and rushed over to my pill container, hoping I could get my regular dosage in my system before the wavelengths messed with me any more and I had a big seizure. I lifted the container to my lips, but it was too late.

The pills missed my mouth and scattered all over the floor, under my bureau and bed skirt I guessed, but I was already busy thrusting my body onto my bed.

I thrust my body with aggression, with an almost illogical violence. I had to get onto the bed to keep me safe, I thought, regardless of whether or not it was injurious to my muscular or skeletal system. Once I reached mid-bed, I dragged myself even further up the mattress.

My strength waned quickly because I was cloaked in what felt like an unending pile of covers. Breathing heavily, I rolled to the left and right, crying out, fighting my constricted ribcage, my nearly paralyzed lungs.

Somewhere along the line, I lost consciousness, yet I continued fighting my body. I only know this because, once the incident was over, I came to on the ground, my muscles even more pulled than before. I was so exhausted that I just lay there, breathing and whimpering.

Eventually, I got up and again plopped on the bed. I drifted off a little. An hour later I decided to get going. I grasped the back of my orange recliner at my bedside, to gauge my balance even though

16
GENERAL INQUIRIES

it rocked under my weight and knocked the floor lamp behind it against the wall. I breathed.

• • •

I WAS FORTUNATE that Mary Grace not only left a general inquiry message on my smart phone, but went on to kindly assist me when I called her back.

I casually observed the photo I had assigned to her number as we talked. I enjoyed her beautiful features: the light blue eyes, the high cheekbones and milky skin, the styled blonde hair that fell to her shoulders. And let's just say I had no difficulty remembering her curves below. She looked great, for sure, but it was more than that with her.

I didn't have to justify myself or prove to her that I was cognizant of my issues. So often, the other nurses would question the truth of my statements, as if I sat at home and made up stories about my seizures, as if I tried to create new symptoms or side effects to complicate their reports.

Perhaps other patients did this. I never really considered it before, but who's to say, with WebMD and the like available to everybody, that Hypochondriacs don't roam the net to seek proof for new conditions?

JOSHUA HOLMES

I briefly told Mary Grace of my most recent seizure, explained that I'd seen better days, but that I would survive, as I had proven repeatedly over the years.

"You are one tough guy," she said.

"I don't know about that, but thanks."

Mary Grace added, "We know you don't want any new meds, we know you aren't willing to try anything else, so we'll just go the non-medicinal route."

"This is why I love you Mary Grace," I ventured. "You are the only voice of reason in this place." I smiled.

She laughed. "So I will go ahead and send a prescription over to the local physical therapy office."

"For my neck, head, and shoulder."

"That's right," she added. "They should be able to help in ways we can't."

"Thanks so much, Mary Grace. It's nice to know someone is holding the fort down there."

• • •

17
SPEED AND MASS

ALTHOUGH MARGE promised that, pending any seizures during league competition, no emergency calls would be made, I wanted my first night to be a smooth experience for everyone. The last thing I wanted was to scare my teammates and spend the rest

ELECTRIC

of my time trying to convince them I was okay, or worse, thwarting alienation.

So, in order to familiarize myself with the environment, to dull the stimuli from the lights and speakers and crowds, I went over to the alley early.

As I walked through the front door I was hit with that leftover smell of cigarette smoke mixed with vacuum cleaner residue. Not a clean smell, but not a foul stench either; just a stale one. Recently turned smoke-free, the alley was far better than it used to be, but still musty and clingy as all get out.

I opted for the smell of grease, and for lunch had a grilled cheese meal with fries and an iced tea at the snack bar, followed by a coffee to wake me up. I sat back in my chair and watched a few die-hard bowlers practice their spins, no concern for the game's cost. I had a private physics lesson right then and there.

From what I gathered, achieving the proper thrust, or balance of speed and mass, was the key to a winning game. The lighter the ball, the faster the die-hard had to throw. The heavier the ball, the less he had to exert himself. It made perfect sense to me.

In the ensuing hours, the alley grew more and more congested. The smell of sweat started to mix with the cigarette, vacuum cleaner, and grease. I felt I adjusted well to the business and odors around me, though. I didn't have an increase in anxiety, lose my ability to speak, experience any auras in my eyes or bubbly sensations in my molars, so I was convinced my first league night would be safe and uneventful in a good way.

JOSHUA HOLMES

I SUCCUMBED TO my impulses that afternoon, bought a new black and gold bowling bag from the Pro Shop that would help the transit from home to alley, and identify my football team loyalties. It might even initiate conversation between my league mates and me.

I blamed the constant promos on the TV screens above the lanes advertising Pittsburgh Steelers paraphernalia. But I'm a sucker for sales, in any case, especially when the branding catches my eye. I justified the purchase by asking, "How often do you buy bowling accessories, Chris, really?"

I transferred my personal maroon, navy, and neon yellow-streaked bowling ball and white, Dexter bowling shoes over to my new bag, and, I had to admit, updates to belongings were nice every now and again. I felt better about myself that night, temporarily anyway.

I'D ALWAYS heard bowling was a blue-collar sport, which in my limited experience, meant it drew a different kind of crowd than I knew. This didn't concern me or anything, since I was looking for something different, but I did mentally prepare myself for any and all possibilities.

And there were a few teams who were definitely more rowdy than others, teams who liked to make a scene and messed with everyone else's head by utilizing the shock factor—yells and expletives at crucial points in the game. It also could have been the beer, I suppose.

But I was assigned to play with a reserved foot doctor and a well-spoken hulk of an ambulance chaser, who both were laid back, carried on good conversation, and also just happened to be amazing bowlers. I had to step back and give myself a pep talk about making premature judgments.

After surviving a harmless initiation prank—a practice throw on a closed lane—and a small scolding from Marge, I seemed to fit in almost immediately. They had a laugh at my expense, but I didn't react much, and I guess they appreciated that I could take their jabs.

I learned my lesson, though. I never tossed a pre-mature practice ball again.

So WHY feet?" I asked over soda and pizza that tasted like better than average, cafeteria food.

"No particular reason," the foot doctor, Burke, responded. "Why any field?"

"I don't know." I said. "I guess you could have helped old people or kids. I was just curious."

"Geriatrics?" Eye roll. "Pediatrics? You haven't given me many options, Chris."

My body still hurt from my seizure at home—especially my right shoulder and back region—so I sat back and enjoyed the talk, as trivial as it was.

"How about Neurology?" I asked.

"Foot pain is where the money is," Burke said to me.

"I can see that," I said. "I get those lifts for my shoes on occasion."

"If he's honest with you, Chris, he'll admit he wanted to specialize in Bunyan removal!" shouted Bender, the ambulance chaser.

JOSHUA HOLMES

The TV above our lane flashed the statement "15-minute practice starts now!" We wiped the grease off of our hands, and pulled out our individual bowling bags, balls, and necessary attire.

"Bunyan removal!" shouted Burke with a grin as he threw a strike. "Is that the best you can do, Bender?"

"I thought it was good," Bender shot back drily.

"Don't come crying to me, Bender, when you've hurt your feet running after a new case."

MY BOWLING average was miserable, to put it mildly, by the end of our twenty frames, but Burke and Bender were nice about it. They both told me not to sweat it and my numbers could only go up from there. Little did they know.

"Get this strike, Chris," said Burke during my last frame. "And we'll do shots." I smiled, tried my best, and threw a wicked spin that missed a strike by inches.

"I'm doing shots anyway," said Bender. And he ran off to the bar.

In the next several weeks my abnormal bowling form would lead to consistent inconsistency and personal frustration. What can I say? I'm a perfectionist. My teammates were amazed by my imperfect stationary stance and my strong curve, but my position and throw inevitably tired me out before my fellow leaguers and kept me around 100 points when Burke and Bender doubled that. So much for the physics lesson.

"Almost had it," they would say. "We'll just hit above our average to offset your score. No problem."

ELECTRIC

I was glad that I had no seizures the first night, didn't even really have to talk about them, and that it was generally a decent opportunity to interact with some neat guys.

The casual nature of the league did help me to walk away, annoyed though I was at my performance. There was a hint of relief, a glimmer of hope that next week I'd improve my average and come through for the team.

• • •

18
CRUNCH

WHEN I heard the crunch of car wheels on the driveway the next morning, my heart started to race. Michael was here, and I was not ready. As I rolled over to put my glasses on and check my phone clock, I muttered, "Oh crap."

I hurriedly pushed my blue-striped covers back, sat up in the darkness, and rubbed my shoulder as I scanned the room for my clothes. My pants were on the floor in the usual place, and I had an assortment of t-shirts at the bottom of the bed.

I guessed he hadn't called me to announce his arrival like I thought he would because it was still morning, and he didn't want to disturb me. He could have forgotten, but I was inclined to give him the benefit of the doubt.

I heard the car door slam outside and the double beep of Michael's horn indicating he had just locked his vehicle. I imagined his walk to the house's side door, and tried to win an imaginary race, to dress, make my bed, oh, and can't forget this, take my medicine, before Michael knocked on the door.

The situation took me back to my college days, when on occasion I accidentally overslept the start of a morning class, and I rolled out of bed and ran, after taking my meds, dreading the inquiring eyes of classmates and the derogatory remarks about punctuality from bitter professors.

I presently threw my covers back into place, put on my pants, pulled on a golf cap, brushed my teeth, and ran to the side entrance just as I heard the first rap on the door.

I unlocked the doorknob and looked up to see a less fit version of my old friend. I noticed he was still a redhead, that he still had unshaven red facial hair. *He's obviously past the honeymoon phase of marriage*, I thought. And then I leaned out the door to see if Linda was around.

"Come on in, Michael."

"Thanks," he said. "And, by the way, Linda couldn't make it. But she says hi."

"I see."

"She did want to, but she had to work."

I picked up the suitcase that rested at his feet, and lugged it to my room, next to the blow-up mattress.

"We'll survive, I'm sure."

"Yes."

"To be honest with you, I usually dine out and relax at the coffee shops. The house is pretty barren, so if you want to stay in, we can watch TV or something. If you want to head out, though, we aren't far from numerous restaurants, two movie theaters, you name it.

SEIZURE

"Well, let's get situated here, and then head out for lunch. I'm famished."
"Ok then," I said. "I am too."

THE LAST lunch we had together was at the Kern Graduate Building at Penn State Main. It was more of a relationship update on Linda and an apology from Michael for keeping me in the dark. So much time had passed. I had earned two collegiate degrees and done freelance work since.

Looking back, that update and apology should have sufficed. At the time, I believe it had. We even went from that sit-down and walked to North Atherton Street to check into the free karate lesson advertised and offered downtown.

I had always been assured that time heals, but in the next several months, I learned time can burn too. I was exposed to the harsh social reality of disability life: a person who was once loyal–Michael, for instance–would turn on me because I was different, perhaps even a threat to normalcy, whatever that was.

I had cleared my head by staying focused on my studies, on my art, and my martial arts routine.But Michael and Linda continued to push me away, altering my lifestyle, and the sincerity of Michael's initial apology was soon in question.

I wondered if Michael even remembered.
"Earth to Chris," I heard. "Snap. Snap."
"Sorry," I replied. "Was just thinking."
"So where are we headed, Chris?"
"Well you're driving, Michael, so it's your call. You know I'm terrible at split-second decisions. When it comes to food."

JOSHUA HOLMES

"Yes you are."

WE ATE at a place called Wonderful Gardens, a Chinese restaurant owned by a man and wife who cooked superb dishes, but who were a bit stingy with their service.

Like the exterior of Bon Ton across the street, there were days when it appeared dark and empty, and I questioned whether or not the place had gone under. ButI was glad to see the neon Open sign flashing in the window this day. I later noticed a door that led to an upstairs loft, where I imagined the couple lived—which meant they could open or close any time they wished, really.

The woman poured us both a cup of tea without a word, and left before we could order. Michael and I just kind of sat there chewing on the free prawn crackers.

We waited a while, ordered our meals eventually. Sometime later, my beef and broccoli arrived, and his General Tso's chicken came out shortly after.

The small talk we used to just ease right into seemed to evade us both. I remembered nights when we impersonated eclectic professors, when we sang random songs into pretend microphones and strummed on air guitars on the couch. It didn't appear we'd be concert-playing anytime soon.

"You like it?" I finally said above a tranquil, Asian version of a modern American radio ballad. It was definitely different from the all-you-can-eat Chinese buffet across town.

I kept the conversation light, told him this restaurant had been a family favorite for some years. We laughed a little about the mural

ELECTRIC

on the wall of a near-naked sumo wrestler grinning smugly, it seemed, at the customers under his watch.

"Not bad," he replied. "Was so hungry, though, I could've eaten my fist."

I told him that if he wanted to do his thing that I could meet up with him later. Or if he wanted me to hang out with him, I could do that too.

"Yeah Chris. Good thinking," said Michael. "Let's meet back at the house tonight."

I was a bit surprised by his choice but a little relieved too. "Alright," I said.

• • •

19
ROUTINE

I SPENT THE afternoon at Starbucks. I know. You don't even have to think it. I frequent this place a lot. Could probably cut back, even. But its been built into my routine for quite some time now, and I happen to accomplish a lot with a computer and coffee in hand.

Call it a schedule, a routine, a focused action, an intentionality—as one pastor put it. In my usual recliner in the back, I had learned so many things, designed so many things, made so many contacts that it just made sense to work here. The results almost justified the money I put out for the ambiance, treats, and lattes.

Though Stone had treated me differently the last time I visited, with a sympathetic kindness I passionately disliked, I hoped for a genuine greeting, and thought he deserved the benefit of the doubt. He deserved another chance.

I was happy that he treated me like any other customer at the register. No specials just for me. He offered me a smile, said hello, asked what I wanted, and told me the barista would have my order out shortly.

I smiled and went my way. *Was that so difficult, now, Stone?* I thought to myself. *Just keeping it real.*

TERRENCE PINCHER, my career counselor, had given me that name and number to call for work, the man pursuing a successful start up, and I had yet to contact him.

I put my cell phone charger on the side table, leaned over and pulled my smart phone from my coat pocket. I called and an automated female voice instructed me to please wait. I would be helped momentarily.

The automated voice continued. She explained the startup was called Synergex, led by Rex Stealth, had been thriving for a number of years, that it was local and listed a number of accolades without stating exactly what they were about. And then there was silence.

As if on cue, Mr. Stealth broke the silence. He answered with a low voice that was half animated, half asleep. "Stealth here. How can I help you?"

"Hello Mr. Stealth. My name is Chris, and Ms. Pincher said you were in need of a designer. Just wanted to make contact and introduce myself."

SEIZURE

"Well, tell you what. We are having interviews at the moment, and if you are willing, we could set up the first phone interview right now."

"Oh. Sure." Abrupt and to the point, but it worked for me. "You give me the time, I'll be ready."

We agreed on a morning call on a day the following week, and I thanked him for his time. I clicked off and put my stuff away. I had to get home to meet up with Michael.

BEFORE HEADING home, I ran by the physical and occupational rehabilitation facility Mary Grace had suggested. If I didn't check into it, I'd never know whether or not my pain could be controlled through this method.

The lobby was small, had just enough room for the six or seven waiting patients. One sat in a wheelchair, one sported a cast, and the rest appeared injury-free, although I knew they had something they needed to fix. I didn't have an overtly visible injury either.

I was glad that the lobby cleared out pretty fast. The facility accommodated quite a number of people at once, staff and patients, and it kept things moving efficiently.

When it was my turn, I was led to a back room and advised by a therapist named Val to fill out a pain assessment form, and to take off my sweatshirt so that she could massage my neck and shoulder, and follow up with an ultrasound.

I was in there for an hour—longer than I expected—and, boy, did I feel achy afterward. I was tight. I would remain so for several weeks until I saw my chiropractor in addition to my therapist.

JOSHUA HOLMES

• • •

20
RED EYES

MICHAEL'S EYES were red when I saw him that night. I noticed he was on the verge of tears at lunch, but I didn't think it necessary to mention. I didn't want him losing his composure in public.

"What's the matter?" I asked, surprised at my friend's display. "Why are you crying?"

"It's Linda, Chris."

"What about Linda?" I sat in a chair across from him.

"I lied to you. She didn't stay home because of work. She left me, Chris." He started crying pretty loudly right then. His shoulders shook as he cried.

"What do you mean she left you?"

"We got into a huge fight. We argued badly and she stormed out of the house."

I had known she was the diplomatic type, addressing issues politically—either via diversion or as an intermediary.

"Could she be at her parents' house?"

"I don't know. It's nearly been a week."

"What was the fight about?"

"Oh. It was something small initially. I didn't comment on her new haircut, and she took it to an entirely different level."

"New level?"

Michael started pacing. "She accused me of not caring about her anymore, of falling out of love, and so on and so forth."

ELECTRIC

"Which isn't true, right?"

"Definitely not!"

"And you don't think you are overreacting?"

"Overreacting!? No. I'm not overreacting!"

"It's worth asking."

• • •

21
KINKS

IT HAD to be frustrating for my physical therapists to work out the kinks in my neck and shoulder only to be informed that it's hard to tell whether or not there's been noticeable improvement because of my seizures.

I wasn't going to lie, though. It would defeat the purpose. While I was willing to admit that they had stopped the jabbing in my head and back, and isolated the pain to the neck and shoulder regions, the ache was still irritating and far from gone.

I had run into similar problems in the past. A seizure between treatments altered everything, and to pin a pain problem on one specific thing when so many muscles and bones were at play was a lost cause. I wouldn't be surprised if I said this again.

I'd almost forced the doctors and chiropractors and therapists to approach my body like an old car. When my parts cracked or when I stalled out, so to speak, I was either lubed up with meds, or gently coerced to turn over for massages, to get my engines going again.

So how is this any different than what other persons with disabilities go through? Only my friends with Epilepsy can relate on the same level. An on-site observer might understand the required degree of determination to push ahead after experiencing an episode.

• • •

22
SOFT SKILLS

REX STEALTH did call me for a second phone interview, but spoke to me with the same level of interest he bestowed on me the first time around. I didn't understand why he even bothered if he didn't intend to hire me.

I went over my academic and professional background, and tried to explain what set me apart. He acknowledged my background, and moved on to other things.

Apparently, Synergex wanted specialists—individuals who didn't work beyond the scope of their specialty—and he wanted to make sure I understood this.

I was surprised because it wasn't many years ago when additional soft skills often made you a better, more qualified candidate in the job market. Now it over-qualified me!

By now, I had found his online profile, the company site that I was trying to improve, and all the additional staff—who just so happened to be family members. Rex sported a long mullet and every kind of non-traditional dress you could imagine. He expressed pride in nonconformity.

SEIZURE

He spoke of casually assembling the existing site on a beach in the Caribbean, and of the fact that he knew it needed work. Perhaps I, if everyone agreed, would be the one to improve the Synergex marketing scheme.

I promised that I would do my best to offer up a feasible design option. He said he looked forward to seeing it.

• • •

23
TIME

MICHAEL'S DILEMMA made me think about time, the measurement of our lives, how he had messed up and just how much I could waste or produce, lose or gain, in a certain period.

Yes, I know, its an abstract line of thinking, but, having seizures, my sense of time alters with each episode, and what I can and can't do in a day or week depends on whether or not my body is functioning physically, or if I'm firing on all cylinders mentally, to use a cliché.

"Do you remember the way they felt?" I randomly asked, referring to Michael's seizures. "Or have you forgotten with time the sensations, the Postictal?"

If one looked up the term Postictal online, the site would loosely describe it as the near-hallucinatory state persons with Epilepsy experience just after a seizure. I was not sure that I totally agreed, but I guess it could vary from person to person.

"It was such a long time ago, dude," he said after a minute. "I sure didn't try to remember them."

"I was just curious," I said. "You know, I have a seizure, and then once it's all over, it seems days have passed, when its really only been a few hours."

"Yes. I know."

"On a different note . . . what are you gonna do about Linda?"

"I don't know."

"Well you aren't just going to let her walk out of your life, are you?"

"I suppose not."

"I don't mean to be rude, Michael, but I think it's about time you found Linda, and tried to make amends."

• • •

24
THE BETWEEN SPACE

IT WAS bound to happen, I thought. I had prayed I wouldn't seize there, but it definitely was a selfish prayer, and I'm pretty sure selfish prayers don't pull as much weight as those aligned with His will. And I was at the alley a lot.

In any case, I was in the small room that housed racks of midweight bowling balls when I took the headlong plunge. I barely missed the racks.

I had felt the seizure starting in the restroom, the fluorescents playing with my eyes, but had no time to react. No time to warn anyone. I didn't even have time to protect myself, to curl up in a fetal position for instance, as I had done many times while attending school.

ELECTRIC

I stumbled forward, through the men's room door, managed a few steps, and then, somehow, twisted my way past the racks, into the group of bowlers sitting at the tall tables drinking beer and teasing each other about tournament scores.

I think the expressed horror, the shrieks, and the generally fearful reactions were heightened by the fact that I dreaded making a scene in a place that was my weekly source of entertainment. I couldn't bear the aftermath.

By now, you understand, from that point on, I was at the mercy of those who found me. Well intentioned or not, they determined the civility or lack thereof. It was no different that night.

THE BETWEEN SPACE is what I called it. The hellish period just after the seizure ended but before I was recovered. It was, in my opinion, the time when I felt most oppressed—confused, scared, exhausted, and out-of-control.

There was something about the alley, as well, that exacerbated the situation. The weight of my oppressive bout was ten times that of any I had previously endured. And it wouldn't end.

Just keeping my head up was tough. My body still dead, motor skills not yet returned, in the Between Space, a smile randomly plastered my face, although it was purely neurologic and definitely not indicative of my true feelings. My body tipped left and then right. Sometimes I landed without injury. Most of the time, I wasn't so lucky.

A doctor might say it was still Postictal, and perhaps some of my symptoms were, but take it from me, the people around me pushed me to the Between Space.

Think about it, my brain was just electrocuted and I was supposed to respond as if it was just another day?

On the one hand, you had the doting caretakers who sat with me, asked me questions, simple and direct yes under normal circumstances, but hard to answer when attempting to function in the Between Space. To complicate things, these caretakers, upon hearing a response often made near delirium, took what I said as normal communication, and asked the same questions over and over until my answer appeased their concerns.

On the other hand, you had the establishment leaders—owners, supervisors, managers, you name it—who made it clear they understood and believed me when I talked, but who, in actuality, were concerned about getting sued; liability their main focus. What got me the most, though, in the Between Space, was that they said, "It's nothing personal, just following procedure," as if, on top of coping with the physical exhaustion and mental strain, I should be able to deal emotionally too, no problem.

There was always that group of onlookers who talked about me and didn't know I knew what they were doing, and had no qualms about loitering over me, adding to my claustrophobia, while, inevitably, there was always one other person whose conscious made him step away and call 911.

AND IT still wouldn't end. Next I had to deal with the cops. Tall and barrel-chested, they drilled me much like a person who had just committed an offense. They even incorporated the stereotypical good guy-bad guy interview techniques.

SEIZURE

"Come here, Chris. Listen up. I understand where you are coming from, but the doctor wants you to go in to the hospital."

"So that's it? I can't decline the doctor's orders?"

"No Chris."

"I just can't believe I have no choice." I turned away, so tired and livid, but out of options.

Simmons ended up on the scene, of course. The one cop I had nightmares about. Call it irony, a divine joke, take your pick, but he stomped over to the "scene of the crime", and took a shrine-like stance, as if his very presence demanded worship.

"You either go with us or in the ambulance," said Simmons. "We won't give you the treatment the EMTs will."

I gritted my teeth, shook my head, and clenched my fist at my side.

What was it with some officers? The posturing that took place was as much due to fear as it was ego. And, again, I understood they were human. But, it seemed, somewhere along the line, they forgot that I was too.

"You can't put your officer persona aside a minute and just take me home? Its right across the street."

"No. I can't do that."

I'll just spare you my thoughts of the medical community. I crawled into the back of the ambulance. Went through their drill. Little by little, just as I had said would happen, I emerged out of the Between Space. By the time I was at the hospital, I told the doctors what would occur, and all three laughed at my procedural knowledge.

While the doctors laughed, I filed a grievance with my insurance company. I didn't see how improvements would occur if I remained silent, accepting the unacceptable, so I made sure my provider knew every oversight and act of misconduct.

I was sick to my stomach for days, it was so traumatizing, my experience in the Between Space. I dreamed about it repeatedly upon leaving the hospital. It eventually passed, however, after I told God I was shot and asked Him to calm me.

WHERE DID healthy self analysis end and destructive self obsession begin? Surely there was a happy medium. Yet I had pondered this for years, longing for an answer.

I asked this because, in that moment, at the hospital again, I knew something had to give: notably, how I, a single, middle-aged guy with Epilepsy, coped. I questioned everything, doubted a ton, until I was too exhausted to continue.

If I examined why anymore, or what was the cause of my condition, the reason behind my pain, and the subsequent events, I was bound to break. I was on the brink, so troubled by the seizure re-runs in my head, and the talks with God that didn't yield reciprocity, as I knew it (that's not to say it wasn't there, because I didn't sense it).

It was one thing to fall back daily on spiritual words of wisdom for consolation, or to use as reminders of what my verbal and active responses should be. It was another to actually apply them and comfortably accept them.

The discomfort of living in discomfort was maddening. Constantly wondering about the purposes of things I might never know was even worse.

If I was honest with myself, though, I had to decide right then and there if I could let everything go. Not just say it. But actually do

ELECTRIC

it. And feel alright with it. And not just some of it, either. It couldn't work that way.

I hated that I had to experience the hell that I did, to the degree that I did, to reach this point, but isn't that so typical of the human experience?

• • •

25
THE RETURN

I DIDN'T EXACTLY know what Michael expected from me. He'd obviously come to York to escape his relational shortcomings with Linda, and was using me as a convenient vacation.

Here I had spent all this time processing the moments he hurt me in college, and it turned out he needed the past to be the past, and wanted me to act as some kind of living tutorial.

Considering how I initially focused on his betrayal, I think Michael benefited most. I didn't torture him over the initial lie, and I feel I commiserated on an acceptable level without guilting him.

On two separate occasions I went on to pose reasonable questions regarding his current state, and even offered up some constructive analysis.

I hoped he didn't intend to stay for an extended period. While I wanted him to fix his problem, it ultimately wasn't up to me, it couldn't be resolved here, and had to be resolved there.

I understood the need to get things out of your system. But life had to move ahead. I only had so much room for a vacating, weepy adult.

And, I admit, if I haven't already, that helping Michael a few days had taken my mind off my pain and my seizures. I temporarily focused on getting Linda back. But it was temporary.

I was both surprised and happy to see—upon arriving home from the hospital—a letter from Michael. He must have sensed that I wanted to help, but also that I didn't want the visit to be long-term. He wrote:

Chris –
Thanks for your hospitality.
You helped me realize what I lost and that I can still save it.
I've decided to go home and make amends with Linda.
Thanks,
Michael

• • •

PART THREE

26
THE MISSION

I TIGHTENED MY schedule over the next couple of months, visiting the rehab facility twice a week, if not more, and stretching nightly before I went to bed. I didn't fill a calendar or anything, but my time was put to good use.

I had to fit my art and design projects in between the appointments, usually on the odd days of the week. We reached a point where we set back-to-back appointments to logistically accommodate me.

I even started eating at the next door grocery store—soup or fried chicken and tea at Weis Markets—so that I could accomplish multiple things on any given day.

JOSHUA HOLMES

On occasion, I even ran into one or two of the therapists who met their spouses for a quick meal over break, which made for a nice yet awkward greeting.

As I mentioned earlier, the discomfort in my head and shoulder would wane with each of the ultrasound treatments, only to return a couple days later. So I made it my mission to overcome the jolts of pain with repetitive exercises.

I became one of their regular fixtures. I got along with everyone, and we all were determined to regain my lost physical capacity. I'd do a half hour of stretching, and a half hour of strengthening.

The battle with my body continued for four months. My bowling game fluctuated, depending on the length of a treatment. I worried things might never improve, but my work and their work eventually paid off.

In the fourth month, the pain-free periods began to grow longer and longer, and my therapist hinted at the possibility of wrapping up my treatment sessions.

I noticed the improvement at the bowling alley, while relaxing at home, in my everyday transportation efforts, and, though I told them they'd miss me, I agreed things were better and could see they had to give my insurance company results.

• • •

ELECTRIC

27
TO CAVE OR NOT

I DISTINCTLY REMEMBER the night I had to decide whether or not it was worth continuing in the league. I must have changed my mind a good ten to fifteen times about walking over to the alley.

I was uptight and overheated, for one, and there really was no guarantee, as there never was, that the evening would be event-free.

I clearly identified my apprehension as a fear or phobia, and I knew the only way to defeat it was to place myself again in an uncomfortable spot.

I tried to question myself as objectively as I would have questioned a client in a counseling session, sparing nothing, so that I made solid decisions.

I had been forced to do this in numerous contexts—professionally and academically—throughout my life, and I surmised this would just be one more instance where I'd have to suck it up, and flush out the emotional wounds later.

I skipped practice and watched TV in my room until I could postpone play no longer.

I picked up my Pittsburgh Steelers bowling bag, put on my shoes and jacket, and made my way across the street.It's hard to explain, but even in that mentally strong moment, I felt emotionally raw. It took several weeks for that feeling to disappear.

WHAT HELPED me integrate back into the league culture so quickly was the fact that Burke and Bender never brought up the seizure. They no doubt had heard about it, no doubt knew I was pretending it hadn't happened, yet they had chosen to leave the subject alone.

The only comparable life event that impacted me so dramatically—aside from my brain surgery—and it was during a fragile stage—was when I became so agitated over standing in front of my class to give a speech that I had to leave the class for the day. My peers rooted for me from their seats, and it really was the only thing that helped me complete the course.

Similarly, Burke and Bender rooted me on in my distress, and I was able to push on. They went ahead that night to tease me about my dating life, or lack thereof, which made me think about Mary Grace, and share my insecurities with the guys.

"Just go for it!" Burke shouted. "You have nothing to lose!"

"Absolutely Nothing!" agreed Bender.

"Call the girl up and ask her out!" Burke laughed and threw a strike.

• • •

28
STEALTH

THE WAY Rex Stealth talked to me originally, part excited, part bored that I was interested in some freelance work, I kind of expected I wouldn't hear from Synergex again, even though Rex suggested a phone interview. He spent all kinds of time singing the company's praises, but even more time emphasizing individuality

SEIZURE

among it's employees, and he no doubt had already seen my extensive online profile, which listed experience to the contrary.

But he contacted me a third time, and asked that I come to an interview at my design school. It felt good to receive an invite, and it was nice to head back to my old stomping grounds as a leading candidate.

I spent the first half of the day catching up with professors and secretaries, checking out new artwork in the gallery, listening to the opinions of new attendees.

I was a bit taken aback when I wasn't the only interviewee; three other candidates sat around a long conference table in the green room, awaiting the same fate.

I had spoken to Terrence Pincher about my reservations concerning Stealth. Eternal optimist that she was, Pincher felt good about the upcoming interview. So much so, in fact, that she picked me up at my house, and offered to take me home after the meeting.

We all had our laptops and designs prepared for a presentation. The web designers were nervous, and us graphic designers were more seasoned. It made it interesting.

We all had been asked to create our own versions of a Synergex website and accompanying ad material. I wasn't that impressed by the two web designers, liked the second graphic designer's ideas, and thought I presented well, considering it wasn't my specialty.

Time would tell whether Stealth wanted to utilize my talents, to hire me. He made clear that he only had enough money to hire one person in the moment.

• • •

JOSHUA HOLMES

29
COURAGE

I MUST HAVE picked up my cell phone and placed it back on the orange recliner near my bed three or four times before I built up my courage enough to ask Mary Grace the question I had feared posing all my life.

My heart raced and my voice quivered whenever I practiced in front of my bureau mirror. I had given up hope that the sound of my voice would change, but I still clung to the possibility that I would experience a greater confidence.

The only thing that encouraged me was my imagination. I could hear Burke and Bender in my head urging me on, telling me I had nothing to lose and everything to gain. And, you know, I couldn't have agreed more.

Before trying again, I breathed deeply, ran my hands through my hair a couple times, looked straight into my reflection, and told myself repeatedly that I could do it. I tried to anticipate a positive response.

I wasn't the type to get rattled by little things. In fact, I prided myself on my strength. And yet this small act, this contact attempt, tested my willpower. Was I up to the challenge?

I called the doctor's office because I knew she'd be there working her tail off, picking up where the triage let up. Right this very minute she was probably standing between the automated double doors, fetching her next patient from the lobby. It took a while but I eventually got ahold of her.

ELECTRIC

She was breathing heavily when she put the phone to her ear. She said, "Mary Grace speaking..."

"Hey Mary Grace! Its Chris."

"Hi Chris."

"So listen... Uh... I was thinking maybe."

Silence. "You were thinking, huh?"

"Yeah. I was thinking, if you are up to it, that maybe we could go out together?" I crossed my fingers and winced.

"Are you asking me on a date, Chris?" I laughed uncomfortably.

"I guess I am."

• • •

EPILOGUE
PUSHING ON

IT WAS that time. The point when all leaguers had to say yes or no to another eleven weeks. After what I had gone through, I initially debated back and forth if I could even return to the alley.

But I had gone back, and I had pushed on. I had even salvaged my initial so-so average. After all was said and done, I could feel good about my accomplishments.

Over the speakers, Marge announced that she would stop at each lane and ask for commitments and contact information. I expressed to her beforehand that I was interested.

I patiently waited my turn. One by one, lane by lane, she took down names and numbers until she was finished.

JOSHUA HOLMES

Burke and Bender told me they intended to move on, that they had had their fill of bowling. That meant I had to find another set of teammates who wouldn't fear me, who could overlook the condition, and would accept me for me.

The thought was one that, at another time, would have crippled me. But as I followed after Marge, I had a good feeling about my new teammates. Marge had paired me well the first time, so I trusted she would do the same again.

She explained as we walked that the league would take a six-week break, that those who chose to return would begin again in May. She said she would use the break time to compile team arrangements, but for me, she had a specific person in mind.

"I think you'll like this guy. He's new to the league, but I've known him a while."

As soon as I saw him from behind I recognized him. His bald head glistened as it did at the coffee shop. Stone was minus his usual attire, the green apron and slacks, and he leaned on a nice bowling bag that replaced the usual broom, but he seemed more relaxed. He wasn't bound by the rules of the workplace. I could relate. The freedom to avoid professional morés was one of the perks of independent work.

I stepped down into the bowling area, and placed my hand on Stone's shoulder.

"Well, isn't this a surprise!"

• • •

STATUS
A NOVELLA

AUTHOR OF SEIZURE
JOSHUA HOLMES

PART ONE

PROLOGUE
INVASION

APPARENTLY, THE call never ended when the phone slipped from my hand to the floor. Instead, the device hit hard, and the impact activated the speaker. My client, Nadine, would hear the second half of the episode through the receiver that settled just feet from where I seized.

It had to be the combination of the low light exhibited from my lamp and the competing light streaks that came at me from every other source. I wasn't stressed, consciously anyhow. But my emotional state had never been a reliable predictor. Perhaps it was that I constantly had to stay alert, had to recognize the seizure could evade me, but also expect it likely could invade me this very instant?

With each passing hour, the likelihood of a scene increased a bit more. And yet, several seizure-free days came and went, causing me to wonder if, just maybe, I would get through the project without frightening anybody. Not to get too melodramatic here, but the uncertainty followed you like a thief anxious to attack and secure a spoil. As Nadine quickly learned.

• • •

"EXTREMELY PLEASED with the proof," Nadine said first. "The book turned out nicely."

For an instant, I imagined her narrow, expressionless face scrunching up in satisfaction, her free hand pulling at her long, brown/blonde-streaked hair.

"That's just great," I said. "That's what I love to hear."

"Better than expected, to be honest."

Even as she talked, I tried to distance myself from any stimuli. I hurriedly turned off the TV. I drew the blinds further. Pushed aside my portable technology. It was a race against time.

"I can't believe we did it!" Nadine continued, oblivious to my situation. "So surreal!"

"Yes," I agreed, now walking to a darker place in the house. "Surreal."

And it was. Up until now, the freelance design job—the consultation, editing, cover creation, and compilation processes—had gone wonderfully, and I hadn't exposed Nadine to any of my condition's antics.

STATUS

"So what next?" she asked. "We talked about making it into an ebook?" That option had been discussed, and my payment for it had already arrived.

My thoughts were getting jumbled. I was struggling to remember the order in which I should act out: Should I sit? Should I walk? Should I talk? I pulled out a chair at the dining table, stopped and put my hand to my mouth, and then internally scolded myself for behaving in a manner that made no sense.

"Ah… Uhuh… I… uh. Ughh." *Here we go*, I thought. The notion of more paid work was exciting, but it wouldn't stop what had started in my head. In more darkness, the electrical storm was spreading, and the next thing I knew, I couldn't reply. The fuse that powered my speech had blown.

My auras were light initially, slight waves, and I did mean to terminate the conversation then, but they grew stronger, into flashes, and, well, you know, inevitably overwhelmed me until I couldn't complete a sentence or even stand upright.

In my final moments of clarity, I grunted and panted, my eyebrows twitching as I attempted to continue the exchange. But it was a lost cause.

There was a heavy pressure in my chest. I took a spill, the burden elevated, and twisted up under the lamp's long cast shadow, I headed into the next phase. A blank phase.

"Chris?"

• • •

JOSHUA HOLMES

I CAME TO what felt like a lifetime later, at an entirely different place in the house, and ironically to the phone ringing.

My forehead, chin, and right hand stung, the signs of carpet burn quickly forming in the three most common points of impact.

In an exhausted frenzy, I got up and stumbled towards the sound. The noise was coming from somewhere near the couch, and last minute I realized from under the cushion.

Phone in hand, I had to rectify the situation, had to allay Nadine's fears; convince her everything would be ok, and that this didn't change anything. Although it would.

I knew I still wasn't in my right mind. Exhaustion and pain had me saying and doing things I never would in my proper state.

"I heard once that seizures shouldn't last longer than five minutes…"

I checked my door lock. Not really sure why.

"I'm sorry," I said. "Really sorry."

"No don't be," said Nadine. "But yeah, I thought you should like call 911 after five minutes."

I then walked to the light switch. Still unsure why.

"No," I said. "Honestly. I'm fine."

"Isn't that like dangerous?"

I was intent on convincing Nadine to forget what she witnessed, but instead slurred an unintelligible response.

"Like couldn't it lead to…What's it called? Status?"

• • •

ELECTRIC

I
SHADES OF BLUE

As I finished at the computer terminal, reading the online, blog article—about a young girl who experienced my usual symptoms and tried blue lens glasses—the following day, reflecting as well on all I'd already tried for my Epilepsy, I asked, "What's one more unconventional treatment?"

Any blue tint I acquired locally would be a substitute for the original, therapeutic color Zeiss Z1 F133 (cobalt). And, according to the article, you could have the real thing applied to a lens, and shipped in from somewhere overseas. But I'd likely see what my personal eye doctor could do.

There was no way I was doing more of the standard: No way I was going through another brain surgery. No way I was doing the Ketogenic Diet. No way I was installing another VNS (Vagus Nerve Stimulator) device in my chest. No way I was going to try another anti-seizure medicine. I was leery about straight up and medical Cannabis use, and the CBD oil—extract or not—didn't assure me in the least. But this? Perhaps.

"Definitely something to think about," the tiny yet vocal assistant said. "Possibly an avenue to pursue in the future, Chris."

"Hopefully not too far in the future."

"Seems the positive strides are here," said the assistant, eager to share her opinion. "Seems that girl is benefitting."

"Well, I've just about tried everything else..."

Still nursing a tension headache from yesterday's bout, it was hard to imagine one hefty investment and a small adjustment to my appearance could improve my day-to-day living. But that was the implication.

"Your doctor never suggested this as an alternative?"

In the thirty plus years I'd consulted doctors, I'd never heard the diagnosis 'photosensitive Epilepsy', much less any fix for the wild sensations I'd endured.

"Never," I said. "You are the first."

Finally at a loss for words, the assistant said, "Wow."

• • •

"**B**LUE ENOUGH for you?" asked Dune, the rail thin, broad-smiling eye doctor, months later.

They were for the time being, after they'd been darkened a second time. I wasn't having near the reaction to outside stimuli, as the red wavelength wasn't impacting me the same.

"Much better," I said. "Incredible. What a difference!"

The first time he'd dipped my glass lenses into the blue pigment, they came out barely tinted, the hue failing to change the amount of auras I was having.

I had a slight reference point, as I'd also ordered and experimented with numerous, cheap, eBay sunglasses in the weeks leading up 'til now with surprising success. Another tentative avenue my neurologist never suggested, by the way.

"You might be onto something, Chris," said Dr. Dune.

STATUS

I nodded and shrugged, mostly because I was unsure. "So far, so good, right?"

• • •

2
COMMUNITY

IF YOU'VE been following my story for any stretch, you'll remember my community in graduate school at Penn State Main had been comprised of my red-headed, best friend, Michael, the debaters, John, Alex, and Linda, the eccentric, local bookstore owner, Sam, the members of the College of Education, Professors Patterson and Love, and attendees of the Kali karate classes I later pursued. Yes, there were a few others who played a minimal role, but that is all.

In the couple years since graduation, the community grew to include Starbucks owner, Stone, Synergex entrepreneur, Rex Stealth, Career Services rep, Terrence Pincher, and bowling league friends, Burke and Bender. It also included additional clients in need of design services. Again, there were a few others. If you didn't already know, you'll soon learn about my history as it relates to this particular account.

In any case, while these new friends weren't close enough to term 'chums', they added another dimension to my 'social life'.

It wasn't easy getting out there, convincing people that—despite the inevitable seizure or two—I was otherwise normal, and like anyone else—with a few exceptions—would contribute to the community as needed.

JOSHUA HOLMES

And I didn't get to this point overnight. Losses and gains in one life stage prepared me for necessary adjustments in the stage to follow. Ironically, it was nearly time to grow my network.

• • •

HANK WAS a lifesaver. At first I only knew him by name, but that changed in time. It wouldn't be long before we had mastered a secret handshake, before we had nicknames for each other, before we were talking about everything under the sun, and I would call him a friend.

After I inquired about the local church's travel amenities, he was approached to see if he could serve as my official driver to and from church and life group, and as the formal introducer to the church community.

I'd gone to a couple other churches that fell short in your usual areas: Travel, worship, and pastoring, all in varying degrees, and I was on the prowl again for a place to grow. Hank would make the transition easier; as easy as it would get, let's say.

Square and short, he was quiet but kind, agreeable to an extent I've never known, and I'm sure my more verbal, more direct personality repeatedly pushed him beyond his comfort zone.

I was living alone, by the way. In York, Pennsylvania, in a complex behind the Queensgate Plaza. On this particular day, he'd stopped by my apartment, and we were now headed across town to a small house on the east end for one of the meetings. My heart was pounding in my chest because of nerves, and I really had to take a deep breath, before introducing myself.

ELECTRIC

I hadn't done the group discussion thing since my college days, and while I enjoyed a healthy debate every now and again, I always had to defeat that clammy feeling right before the big moment.

But, generally speaking, I was eager and grateful for the opportunity to broaden my horizons and contribute to a new support system.

"So tell me what this is like," I prompted from the sedan's passenger seat. "Deep, surface, a romping good time?"

"Sure."

"All of the above?"

"Sure."

"Young people? Older people?"

"Sure." I took that to mean a bit of both.

"I assume I should moderate my sarcasm."

"Probably."

"You mean they won't accept me for the stranger that I am?"

"They might," said Hank. "Or they might not."

I laughed at this, and could really only wait and watch as it unfolded before me.

• • •

3
THE DATE

"YES," SAID Mary Grace. "I'd love to."

Those words kept repeating in my head. I suppose I'd spent such a long time brooding over asking her on a date and the possible outcomes, that when she answered quickly and favorably, it caught me by surprise. The build up was completely erased.

"Yes?" I repeated back to her. "Just like that?"

"Just like that," she said. "Unless you want me to say no, and twice as slow…"

"I think I'll take it as is," I said. "Thank you."

I'd already spent a long time wondering about her possible baggage and her thoughts of our relationship, so I put that aside. Still in a state of shock, though, it took a few tries to process what I'd heard, to think logically and on all cylinders.

If my former bowling league teammates, Burke and Bender, were here now, they'd be offering congrats and slapping me high five. They'd encouraged me to make this call for about a year.

"I'm still on duty, here at the office, Chris," said Mary Grace. "Did you have a place in mind?"

I was so surprised that I failed to cite a place to dine. I could have mentioned Ruby Tuesdays or Cracker Barrel, thinking on it after the fact. But instead: "Well Mary Grace," I said. "Anywhere you like."

"Why not the new place just a little ways from Wellspan Neurology?"

Nice and close to work, I thought. *Not a bad idea. Not bad at all.*

• • •

THE DATE was no doubt a victory—at the Stone Grille & Taphouse in the St. Charles Way Plaza, too, but ask me to recount the night in its entirety, and I'd probably do the evening a disservice.

STATUS

It was a busy place, but an open one. Plenty of room for a couple to interact, and, surprisingly, quiet; easier than say, Texas Roadhouse, to converse.

Conversation was easy for me, and I sensed she felt the same, as she didn't seem to be rushing to leave. She savored her cup of wine, and then continued comfortably discussing another topic.

"So how was your day?" I said somewhere along the line. "Good, I hope."

"Yes, my day was good," she said with an inviting smile. "Thanks for asking."

I bowed my head, and said, "Chris here, at your service."

"You always were a good listener."

"Thank you. Now your day... Tell me about it," I said. "If you like, of course."

"Helped several patients today... updated medical records... confirmed some refill requests...made several calls to insurance companies for the neurologist."

"Any shakeups within the nurse triage?"

"No controversy to speak of there, although I have to correct their mistakes all the time, like I always did."

"As far back as I can remember, you were the only one who came through in that regard."

"How about you, Chris?" asked Mary Grace, crossing her legs. "Was your day a good one?"

"It was," I said. "Routine freelance consulting work... Helping clients publish and advertise...designing websites here, book covers there. A bit of this. A bit of that."

JOSHUA HOLMES

Rex Stealth—previously mentioned head of start up Synergex—had given the web design job for which I interviewed to someone else, and ever since, I'd worked alone exactly as I told Mary Grace.

"Anything new to speak of in your life?"

I tried to keep it casual, offering a suave smile. Beyond that, I didn't offer anything about my seizure numbers, anything regarding medicine, or anything regarding condition-related injuries from which I was always recovering. And she didn't push for particulars. Yes, it was my life, and subsequently difficult to avoid, but, still, it was hardly romantic.

I did manage to say, "Professionally, it's been consistent. And personally, I'm still getting used to the new glasses. Other than that, though, I'm trying to stay active. To be productive. To get involved at a new church."

I don't remember saying much else. However, I couldn't forget how terrific she looked, that's for sure. No one could beautify curves beneath medical attire, blue eyes, and mussed up, long blond hair quite like her. Or genuinely present a grin that stirred something so strongly inside me. It was all good.

The food was good too. Mary Grace went the healthy, green route with a large, fancy salad, while I went the usual, less-than-calorically acceptable route with a meat and potato dish topped off by an incredible dessert.

While we both enjoyed the evening tremendously, and I left feeling great about the progress we made, I reminded myself to keep it in perspective:

ELECTRIC

One date was simply that. It was an achievement to enjoy, and nothing to take lightly, but something to assess and build upon. That is, if Mary Grace and I were to ever amount to anything long-term.

• • •

4
MANAGE

I WAS STARTING to forget the things that I valued so much about my friendship with Michael, and it worried me. Palm to my forehead, I unsuccessfully tried to recall what I seemed to be losing. Was it simply a memory deficit due to head trauma? Or was it something more permanent?

When it mattered, I couldn't have valued anything more, or even imagined valuing someone else to a greater extent. But as with many things in life and over time, my values changed, and others were replacing that empty spot inside.

I was starting to make a habit at night of recollecting my younger years, reassessing the things that satisfied me then, considering the power of said things now, and how I currently dealt with Michael's growing absence.

It wasn't like I had to re-learn how to adapt or anything. I'd repeatedly picked myself up after those closest to me took advantage of my loyalty and friendship. I suppose I had to take responsibility, as—like so many—I'd allowed it until I grew weary of the same patterns repeating themselves.

JOSHUA HOLMES

I was perfectly content to acknowledge my mistakes and imperfect humanity, but I also remembered my strength and resilience. I worked hard to accrue them. And, to an extent, I had to rely on them.

I managed when the couple broke their ties with me over Epilepsy, when out of fear of my condition they voiced their desire that I attend the concert alone, managed when they quit and abandoned me at school because they were so in love, and later when they had a private wedding without me. I managed to forgive him when he used me to escape and return to Linda when he argued with her and was ready to make amends. And frankly, despite what anyone claimed, I would manage any other obstacle that arose out of this drama.

• • •

5
AESTHETICS

AFTER YEARS of enduring nearly all seizure types, I was used to people staring at me out of pity during the Postictal phase, but I hadn't yet grown accustomed to people gawking because of an aesthetic change.

In fact, I think of everyone in my family—although I enjoyed shopping, collecting golf caps, and generally looking nice—I was least concerned about keeping up with the current trends and achieving a particular style.

STATUS

I was content to live constructively in the shadows, to accomplish things without notice, to maintain a simple yet comfortable routine in leisurely attire beyond the spotlight.

Since sporting my new, blue lens glasses, however, I had one guy compliment me on the color, a few girls suggest I looked like a Hollywood type (which I still didn't get), and numerous others gaze skeptically at me, as if I was a lost youth searching for identity in eyewear.

With a nod, I usually said, "They're for my seizures." And then I secretly enjoyed their squirms, how they attempted to mask their surprise and embarrassment.

The funniest ones, though, were those who watched me a long time, almost said something, hesitated, and then pretended they were looking at something else entirely. Nine times out of ten, they knew how obvious they were, and still hoped the guy with blue glasses would somehow miss it.

I never did.

• • •

THE SKEPTICAL looks were a small price to pay if my seizure numbers decreased. I was told multiple times by my neurologist, I was just one of those cases that couldn't be fixed. So the slightest improvements were noted.

For several months, I followed my patterns and saw a minor decrease. But I also saw a trade off. How so, you wonder? Well, I realized I had fewer, severe Grand Mals, but more auras that turned generalized and stopped in a different area of the brain, leading to strange seizure types. This sometimes enhanced my post seizure obsessions and headaches, yet increased the speed at which my lost motor skills returned to me.

Were these changes improvements? Or just moderate differences? I didn't know. So I didn't commit to a position, one way or another. I wasn't one to say life was better or worse because it was easier or more difficult.

Regardless, I was hopeful.

• • •

THE CLIENT who witnessed my seizure on the phone, Nadine, was still shaken our next meeting, but intrigued by the aesthetic change.

"I've heard of people with migraines using different colored glass lenses. Do they really help?" said Nadine. "I know you said it probably wouldn't ever happen, but that one day, you know, I still thought you were close to Status."

"I've noticed some changes for the better," I said. "To an extent, I think."

"How'd you hear about that?" I told her of the blog article, and then redirected the conversation to her published book.

"I've sold fifteen so far!"

Nadine was benefiting from the recent interest increase in New Age thought. For some reason, the vagaries of the philosophy drew a lot of curious idealists.

"Awesome!" I said. "Nice way to start!"

ELECTRIC

"Yeah," said Nadine. "If you'd have told me I'd earn that much in my first month, I'd have said, 'no way!'"

"And yet here we are!" I said. "Congrats again!"

• • •

6
INTERVIEW

ONCE SITUATED on the couch in the living room of the tiny house where the church community gathered, and after Hank meekly introduced me to everyone, I withstood several rounds of kind yet rigorous interview questions, all in attendance trying to pick away at the personal background that I didn't just hand out to anyone.

I apparently hadn't hidden my discomfort too well, as the five or so couples seemed to enjoy the apprehension and brevity with which I offered my history.

Hamilton "Ham" Reed—a large, single man who sported a grayish, bowl cut and long sideburns—quickly became the center of attention and lead interviewer. Right away, he disclosed an unending list of work problems that plagued him in manufacturing, how emotional he was about it, and then through tear-riddled eyes inquired about my own state of affairs.

Lanny Galt, a perpetually happy, dark-haired, trim, executive type in slacks and a suit coat shared a corny, 'why did the cat cross the road?' joke a guy at the office told him. And then he said, "Yes Chris. Tell us more about yourself!"

JOSHUA HOLMES

"Yes," chirped his small and equally fit, high-pitched, white-haired wife, Leah Galt, who exuded several, canary-esque qualities. "Tell us!"

"Not much to tell, frankly," I said. "My life is rather uneventful."

Sylvia Fanning, a single portly woman with red, close-cropped hair, and a masculine jawline, listened with a scrutinizing expression. Her only response was: "Hum." I didn't try to read into it, because not only was she the hostess, but also because the story, I'd discover, was that her social contribution didn't sweep any further.

There was one other person there: A visitor named Foster Monroe also interested in experiencing a new life group. He looked to have about ten years on me, perhaps in his mid-forties. He had wispy, greyish-brown hair, combed back, near black eyes, rubbery skin, and generally seemed tired. He turned out to be a truck driver, and the only one who said nothing.

I honestly didn't realize how important I found keeping things to myself, until I was poked and prodded with the finger tip, and forced to explain my life situation. When all was said and done, I reluctantly recognized that I begrudged the position.

I kind of resented the dress code, as well. I didn't dress super conservative, but I didn't go very liberal, either. Tan jeans and a Polo shirt the combo, it was one that passed at a nondenominational church for formal/casual, and at a place like this was probably bordering on messy.

Granted, I didn't want to alienate anybody. My Epilepsy did that for me. However, I didn't want to invite anybody into my personal space via some false persona.

STATUS

But yeah, I breathed deeply again and braced myself for more. I hadn't shared the intricacies of my world in a while. Things picked up after we finished with the customary worship, study questions, and prayer time.

"When were you saved?"
"When were you baptized?"
"Where'd you go to high school?"
"Where'd you go to college?"
"What do you do for a living?"

In slacks and a plaid, button-down, Hank sat next to me—dressed more conservatively, and closer, I imagined, to the accepted, unspoken dress code—in silence, and quietly listened to the litany of inquiries, unless he was otherwise addressed. Every now and again they'd ask him a question, so as not to appear partial. And Hank always obliged with a nod or light, verbal acknowledgment.

The list went on and on. I tried to offer enough information to content them, but abstain enough that I wouldn't have to dig myself out of a pit, whatever it might be.

I was always told that, with practice, relief would come. But it never did. I hadn't expected to experience discomfort to the degree I did, yet—despite constant prayer—I would, and for a number of months at that.

• • •

7
ROADBLOCK

I'M NOT sure what I was thinking, but I guess I didn't foresee a roadblock so soon after my solid date with Mary Grace. I did give myself a pep talk—a reminder that it had only been one dinner—but I suppose I had confidence in our history, and what we were. Now all I could do was wonder, What exactly did that mean?

I had started getting comfy in that warm sense of belonging, too. As if I'd somehow—after such a long time—achieved a different level of overall acceptance, or self-pride. Deep down, I knew it had been premature.

Perhaps I should have assumed my seizures would still be a big issue for her. Perhaps I should have known the relationship wouldn't develop without others attempting to infringe upon it. Perhaps I should have expected competition. A million other thoughts crossed my mind when I saw the pillar of a man opening the building door for her from afar.

What made it twice as bad, though, was the bright smile on her face. No sign of guilt or betrayal in her eyes. No indication the guy was a friend or family member. I remember thinking, *If I don't do something about this right now, all my work could go down the drain, and my dream girl might just slip away from me.*

• • •

THE "ACCIDENTAL" run-in was orchestrated in such a way that I was able to gather some quick information, and interrupt the

ELECTRIC

nice time Mary Grace was obviously having with Mr. Perfect. Not that I was a blatant date wrecker, but I couldn't allow for this to happen right in front of me!

I had stopped by the office—one lone, rectangular building comprised of a central waiting room, sign-in center, an adult wing, children's wing, and a neurosurgery wing—to express what a nice time I'd had, when I was planted with an eyesore if there ever was one. I got a close look at my competition, listened to the tone of his voice.

By the time I made it over to their area, they were loitering around what I assumed was his red, sports car, laughing and flirting.

Flirting, I'd say, like a pair beyond familiar with one another. Too familiar for my taste, especially since it suggested a level of mutual security I thought was only exclusive to Mary Grace and me.

Neither Mary Grace nor Mr. Perfect appeared to be in a hurry. But I had made that same observation when she was dining with me. Seeing her behave similarly with someone else made me question many, if not all, judgments I made the other night, and generally disgusted with the dating process.

Mary Grace noticed my approach, and said, "Oh great. Let's get out of here." This from the same supportive beauty who usually consoled me when doctors were rude.

What a difference a day or so made! She embraced my arrival so nicely before. Now she was eager to escape me!

"What do you mean?" said Mr. Perfect, annoyance evident on his face. "Thought we were having a good time."

"For sure," said Mary Grace at a higher decibel, I assumed, to convince him. "But we have company."

Mr. Perfect—in impeccable, physical shape, mind you—tensed up, and looked around, eager, it seemed, for a fight.

"You want me to take care of him?" *Just my luck*, I thought. *The guy wants to take me out.*

"No," said Mary Grace. "Let's just get out of here. I'll tell you about it later."

The car doors slammed and the tires squealed as they sped by me. I hadn't exactly ended the date, but at least I forced them elsewhere.

• • •

8
PAST & PRESENT

I THINK I'VE said it before, but if ever you had to enhance drama in a movie scene, you inevitably slowed things down and added a classical piece or ballad in the background. Subsequently, the scene would always improve tenfold.

I mention it because I could use a little enhancer right here, but I will avoid embellishments and attempt to address my past and present as I have in previous writings: Succinctly and with purpose.

I mean, really, how easy was it to drift back in time to places in life that were enjoyable? And, alternately, how easy was it to recall equally tough times? If you didn't reign in your focus, let me tell you it was pretty darn easy.

On my bed again, I fell back into my routine. I tried to bring up some of the good memories I had with Michael (and they were there), although it proved to be difficult.

STATUS

It was kind of like pushing aside and meandering through rows of glass cups in a cabinet for a favorite mug just out of reach. You wanted your arm to make its way through multiple goblets for a shot at one in particular. But you weren't really thinking about the utter mess you could make with one unexpected tremor, or with one wrong touch if any cup would tip over. A few positive memories surfaced as I bumped into a few unwanted ones.

For instance, a few of the times Michael had loyally assisted me in my Postictal period, the times he had waited for my return without making me feel ashamed (as a kid, mostly), the nonchalance with which he spoke of my seizures, returned with a clarity nobody with Epilepsy would purposely dismiss.

And certain moments popped up: Building forts together as teens, occasional shared boyhood crushes, some of our mutual excitement over heading to college together, finishing off especially difficult semesters after months of anti-seizure drug experimentations gone awry.

But like I mentioned, it seemed the act of recollection was becoming more of a chore than a luxury. Flashback was used so frequently as a filler tool in movies today that it seemed people forgot—in real life—it could be torturous.

Covers pulled to my chin, darker instances I either wanted to totally disappear, or show one final time in their entirety, came and went in patches.

How long would the instances return in patches? Would there come a time they'd fade completely?

• • •

# 9
COLOR SHIFT

PROBABLY MORE than the staring from others, was the evident color shift of my entire world. You can't really appreciate the impact of the color red, until it's omitted from your spectrum.

The intensity with which all things crossed my visual field wasn't as strong now, but altogether different. Lighter and duller in most instances, but brighter in others.

The reality of my condition was that I could potentially fall victim to any light wave at any moment. If I was hit too many times, or from the wrong angle, I could drop instantaneously.

Some days, behind the glasses I felt protected from any and all light forms, while other days I felt unusually vulnerable to the light. I wasn't sure, but I didn't think there was a psychological element to this like there was with the VNS devices (which I'd also had installed in my neck and chest for a number of years, to no avail).

I'd always dealt with aura-filled days that visually impacted me one way or another: Differently in the past, but still frequently. The world immersed me like a cloak, the sensation felt as if I'd entered a separate plane, and color constantly overcame me.

So I didn't miss the color at all. Like light, it could be friendly, but was more often my enemy. Blue things were especially blue, green things particularly green, and 'warm' things instead a dark yellow. When I was working with color—digitally or manually—I had to remove the glasses, so I'd see the colors in their true hue, or so I'd see a red shirt, let's say, as cherry instead of coral.

ELECTRIC

• • •

EVEN AS I adjusted to the color shift, I'd pushed on with the creation of the ebook version of Nadine's New Age autobiography.

I didn't consider myself an expert in the ebook development area at all, but still trustworthy and adept; I had noticed that people looking to hire independent designers/consultants like myself would pay extra to finish off the project details, so I taught myself how to prepare manuscripts for .mobi and .ePub editions, otherwise known as iBooks (and others) or Kindle books, to add another dimension to my list of offered, freelance services. Evidently, it was a good move.

It was a redundant process. The human eye never caught all mistakes the first time, so—even when I felt good about an edit—I knew I'd find something in the next round.

At my dining room table, in front of my life size canvas painting of two embracing zebras, I explained this to her.

Fortunately, I had successfully assured Nadine I didn't anticipate achieving any degree of Status, and our talks hadn't strayed much. She did start by tapping her eyebrow, and asking, "Have the shades done the trick?"

"Sort of," I said with a smile. "Thanks for asking.

"Here's a glance at the near-final version," I said, changing topic and turning my computer screen in her direction. "I noticed a few things that need altered, but, generally speaking, this is what the product will look like for your readers."

The book had the cover and meta-data there, the title page, copyright, the Table of Contents, and the rest of the interior in proper order.

"I'm blown away!" said Nadine with a look to the ceiling and a clap. "My own ebook!"

"Feels good, huh?"

"Beyond words," she said. "Beyond words."

"Now to sell it!" I said.

• • •

10
FINDING COMFORT

I WAS ABLE to find a little comfort in the tail end of the church group's meeting, believe it or not. The formal, interactive lesson part (which never felt natural to me) had finished, and we all made our way out into the dining room, where a nice selection of snack foods and sweets were arranged, and the participants threw their traditional verbiage to the wind, and conversed with me in a more modern manner that I better understood.

Conversation over dessert moved into less personal territory, into the casual talk most men thrived amidst: Big sporting events, recent commendable movies, new restaurants to try, sometimes politics. The focus seemed to shift off of personal accomplishment—or lack thereof—and onto topics of little interest, topics that wouldn't arise again if any of us could help it.

Hank and I carefully leaned over our plates, crumbs landing right where they ought, and snacked politely before the broad, blinds-covered, encasement window with lengthy, white curtains.

STATUS

"Pretty good," I said, pointing to a brownie with a plastic fork. "Can't remember ever having eaten such a moist brownie!"

"Yeah," said Hank, stuffing his mouth.

"Delicious."

"In fact," I said, getting up. "I think I'll have another."

Upon my return, Hamilton Reed pulled up an ornate, wooden chair, trying miserably to place it without scratching the floorboards. He was sad again, looked to be near tears from another work tragedy, old water stains already etching his cheeks.

Lanny Galt jovially observed the man, and good naturedly said, "Rough week, huh Ham?" Following

Reed's sad confirmation, he tisked his tongue and nodded with what appeared to be pure understanding.

"You've said things were especially hard. Surely it will get better."

Leah Galt emphatically agreed, dashing about the room, head bobbing and full of positivity, until the other women in the group supported her and followed suit.

Sylvia Fanning raised her chin—perhaps a bit higher than normal—to note the moment's importance, and hummed her regular, noncommittal chord.

Foster Monroe wasn't there to add anything, but nearly everyone else nodded in agreement. I didn't doubt the legitimacy of their attempts to show empathy. "It always does, Ham."

I was starting to see who were introverts and who were outspoken, who were pacifists and who leaned aggressive. If Reed needed a regular encouragement, both Galts needed a few extra forced laughs, and all Sylvia Fanning wanted to do was hum, I could handle that. It was hard to know, harder to imagine, but perhaps things would become easier.

• • •

11
CAT & MOUSE

THE MAIN question I had to answer was a concrete, yes or no query—as most of mine were—and yet it was just as tough, if not more so, to answer than some of the others. Did I really want to participate in a cat and mouse chase to win back a lady (Mary Grace) whose heart I'd obviously lost? Did I really want to exhaust my emotional energy on someone who might not reciprocate with me? Risk having a seizure? Or was it time to walk away? Sounded easy enough to pick one or the other, right? Wrong.

There was this wonderful thing called the "male ego" that I was trying to preserve. To say yes or no to one choice, was to give up control of the other. Which was hard for everyone, even if they didn't admit to it.

Ever the diplomat, my first inclination was to look at both options, and consider if and how I might be able to do a little of one or both. Why not cut myself a break, and attempt to make a taxing debate simpler?

When all was said and done, however, I was not the type to give up on anything, regardless of the physical or mental consequences. It was one thing to put forth the effort and fail, and as a result, stop pursuing a given direction. It was something entirely different to

ELECTRIC

embark on something else without having even first tried the original path. Because I would feel wrong if I didn't attempt to woo Mary Grace back, after much consideration, I decided to try.

• • •

TRY HARD as I might, the task didn't decrease in difficulty. In fact, I'd venture to say the mountain I had to climb grew steeper, as it usually did before it peaked, leveled out, and finished its descent.

I wished it were a stretch to say it felt Mary Grace and Mr. Perfect were everywhere, but it wasn't. York County was like the larger, renowned college towns in that you could run into people when and where you least expected. And those of us who kept busy could share the same activity on any given day or night.

The next time I ran into them was one of those days. It was coincidental, believe it or not, but no less devastating. I almost shouted in front of everyone, "Just kick me in the gut, why don't you?" Last minute, I refrained.

I was getting a movie ticket at one of the grey, automated stations at the big cinema here, called Frank's Theatre (a place I frequented almost every weekend, by the way), when I spotted them over near the flashy arcade.

I couldn't look in the arcade's direction too long, as the strobes, explosions, and general commotion promised to trigger and strengthen my auras, but I looked long enough.

Mary Grace and Mr. Perfect were with another couple—on a double date, perhaps?—more clingy and overtly social than before. You know how juvenile young people with crushes can behave.

They kind of acted like that. Thing was, Mary Grace and Mr. Perfect weren't so young anymore; my age, to be fair.

Mary Grace looked away as quickly as she could, but not before giving me that oh so obvious nonverbal: *not now, Chris. Please not now.* Which I noted with resentment.

I went to my movie, tried to release the experience, and enjoy the film. But it was a waste of money and a moot attempt, because I was so hurt. I had a deep ache in my chest that just lingered.

The one thing I'd consider later was that she'd seen that hurt expression on my face and in my body language before, in several contexts too, and reassured me for years! Yes, in recent days she'd chosen Mr. Perfect, but would that last? Would she be able to dismiss the person in whose welfare she'd so kindly and thoroughly invested?

• • •

12
BRIEF GLANCE

THE BRIEF glance at the small, black, Mr. Coffee, four-cup coffee maker in the far corner of my kitchen, at the rear of the brown, Formica counter, earlier this morning instigated a slew of images that, until several hours ago, were either locked away or well on their way to exiting my memory bank. If I had a choice, I preferred an exit to imprisonment.

STATUS

And to think I'd bought the name brand contraption on sale the day before to serve as a pick-me-upper, to awaken me for positive reflection.

In any case, these revived images were scattered, yet vivid enough that they assimilated into quick scenes specific to certain deteriorating events and places including my old friend Michael.

I assumed the venture into my current kitchen, and across the white, linoleum floor to the coffee pot reminded me of the Penn State Main graduate school kitchen of old, where I'd spent several an aromatic hour sitting with my friend, eating dinner, preparing for his debate club, or for Monday Night Football.

Vivid enough, but not vibrant, per se, there was joy and laughter and anticipation, but there also was pain and a lasting sting at that table that didn't necessarily exist with explanation. As was the case for most people, and their many life events and/or stages. I will add that—directly or indirectly—my condition, Epilepsy, normally was at the heart of my own, but I'm sure you've already picked up on that.

In my room before bedtime once again, a wide scope of feelings gnawed at my psyche. I tossed and turned, twisted in my sheets, sunk deep within one of my two pillowcases, agitated as the sequence—or lack thereof—just fed the disorder, and I didn't have enough control or desire to retain the images.

Perhaps it was a sign. Perhaps the friendship was presently doing more damage than good. Perhaps that was why a Mr. Coffee could trigger something disturbing; why, sub-consciously, memories were daily slipping away.

JOSHUA HOLMES

• • •

13
LASTING

DAYS SEEMED to be lasting longer since donning the glasses. It's not a complaint. An observation of something I had never considered previously, but a fact that clearly impacted my day's success.

In other words, though seizure meds still made me drowsy, I wasn't tiring as quickly, because the blue lenses soaked up my enemy. And I was able to work before my computer—stare and create—and avoid overstimulation to an extent I'd never before known.

I'd be remiss if I didn't add that a suggestion to adjust my computer screen's color settings led me to seek out additional alternatives, modify light strength, and also lengthened my day.

With each positive adjustment, however, there was a caveat. I could work longer, yes, but I still could overdo it (which I did more often than I talked about). There were days I timed it perfectly, and made it 24 hours without incident; and other days, when I'd work nine or more hours instead of eight, and—bam!—I'd have a series of hard Grand Mals.

I had to more closely regulate the degree to which I pushed myself, I supposed. I'm hardly advocating regulation beyond this context; just saying, I was learning a little extra attention could benefit my overall health.

I'd heard two general responses to my musings: "It's nice to see you say that. Now follow your own advice!" and also "Everybody's got to work in tough conditions! You're no different!"

ELECTRIC

It really was a balancing act. I wanted to agree with the latter sentiment, but was still attempting to preserve my body, to last longer if you will.

• • •

BY GIVING Nadine a glimpse at the ebook to come, I allowed myself to break the final stage of creation into smaller development segments. I worked long hours on the refinements, but I intentionally lessened the load.

I opened and worked on my laptop for three hours. Then I shut it down and pushed it aside. Then I opened it, worked, and shut it from time to time, just trying to responsibly control my environment, to be more conscious about my limits.

Nadine took her time, I noticed, but finally called me back on my cell. During conversation, the original seizure she witnessed came up here and there. She did her best to act like it was a thing of the past, but I knew she was well aware it was not, that it was my norm. It was still an experience no one in his or her right mind would want to have happen again, and I was sure its hypothetical re-emergence haunted her.

"Oh take your time," said Nadine. "Sales are still good, and I'm getting good feedback from everybody."

"I just might take you up on that."

"Whatever you do," she said. "Don't stress over it."

I wished I could control that, and quietly longed for the ability.

"That's the goal," I said. "Now to accomplish it."

"Life's too short." *Wasn't that the truth?* I thought. *Just like the space between deadlines.*

"I'll do my best," I said. "I promise."

• • •

14
ICEBREAKER

THE NEXT group meeting, Hank and I didn't have to make our way as far east as we'd gone the previous visit. If I had to guesstimate, I'd say we drove half the distance to get to the Galts' house, which was larger and more conducive to the group in attendance.

The place didn't fall into any particular style category. It was spacious and multi-tiered, had an ideal kitchen to snack in, and had a nice CD player for worship time.

I had left the last time accepting that each attendee had individual needs, that a few would require a little extra attention, recognizing things weren't easy, but hoping for simplicity.

I imagined the right life group would fit me like a snug shoe. It would take a little bit to break it in, would initially feel tight, the laces pulled taut, but with a good icebreaker, with some interaction, would accommodate me as I stretched myself and moved ahead.

• • •

"OUR ICEBREAKER," said Leah Galt. "Was 'Describe a time you were afraid, and how you defeated the fear'."

STATUS

Lanny Galt laughed at this, and said, "I haven't done this a lot, but I went to one of these survivalist camps to zip line... Scary, but I had to have faith in the specialists."

"One time that stands out to me is when I had to speak in front of all the ladies at church," said Leah Galt. "I looked beyond the crowd at the back wall."

Ham pushed away tears and started to choke up. "I was really frightened when I was called into the boss's office at work. I just had to hold it all in."

Sylvia Fanning raised her chin and let loose a deep-throated hum.

"How about you, Chris?" asked Leah. "Any good stories?"

I had hoped my coping threshold would sustain me, and I'd easily open up to my group, and yet I still held back at first. What was that adage? You couldn't get in trouble for saying too little?

Foster Monroe was again missing and unavailable to save me. Man, I wished he had. With watchful eyes, the couples guilt-tripped me into trying.

"I suppose I felt afraid when I seized in public," I said. "Since I was basically a dead weight afterwards, I guess I just had to hope the EMTs and Cops knew what they were doing."

• • •

15
HOME TURF

YOU MIGHT wonder how I could still have feelings for and be attracted to Mary Grace after seeing her with Mr. Perfect twice already. I know I had wondered that, and racked my brain and heart over it, especially the third time we crossed paths.

I concluded that, of course, she was physically attractive (which always helped), but beyond that, it was more about a sense of attachment. She'd been with me in so many instances, particularly as it dealt with seizure recovery and healing, that it was the possibility of her disappearance from my present and future that spurred me on, regardless of the dire circumstances.

You could say the last sighting was on my home turf, too. Any place within walking distance of my apartment could technically fall into that classification. But more than any other, Suburban Bowlerama was at the front of the list.

Starbucks manager, friend, and relatively new, league teammate, Stone, and I—like most weeks—were finishing up our session on lane six, doing our best to seal up a first place spot, even as Marge, the alley owner's wife, attempted to prematurely usher in a new group of bowlers.

I was this close to offering her a piece of my mind about my right to play a game at my own pace when I bumped into Mr. Perfect and Mary Grace, who clearly seemed to have dismissed me.

"Round of drinks on me," shouted Mr. Perfect. "If Team Mary Grace wins!"

I lost my train of thought when I looked at Mary Grace. I caught her in mid-laughter, a toothpaste commercial smile and a sparkle gleaming from ear to ear, though she meant it for Mr. Perfect, whose arm onto which she tightly clung.

ELECTRIC

"And I plan on winning!" she shouted, punching the air, parting a wisp of smoke from the nearby bar, Alley Oops. "Winning big!"

For a minute we locked eyes, and I thought I glimpsed a hint of remorse. But it quickly faded when she returned her attention to my nemesis.

"Best bowler I know," said Mr. Perfect. "And she's mine!"

"And I'm thirsty for a Bud!" added Mary Grace. "Watch out!"

These statements jarred me from my trance. *His?* I thought. *Did he really just say that? And did she just let him?*

Keep in mind, I was relatively new to the courting thing. It hadn't been long ago I was a regular to the friend zone, not that long ago I was still working up the nerve to ask anyone out. Even more recently, I'd courageously asked Mary Grace, specifically, and formally wined and dined her. Now I had to pick up my pants (did I really just use that cliché?), and convince her I was the better candidate? Time was passing, and I didn't see any other choice.

If only it was as simple as handing over a record of accomplishment, or a list of personal attributes I knew would compliment hers. If only.

Yet I knew it would take more.

• • •

16
NIGHTMARE

IT WASN'T your typical nightmare, yet a nightmare nonetheless. There wasn't a death scene, homicidal or suicidal or natural. There wasn't a hijacking scene. There wasn't even a scene that included disappointing a significant other. There wasn't a traumatizing dispute, which always seemed to arise. Even worse, however, there was absolutely nothing to latch onto.

To complicate matters, the recollections were also clipped, like the ones before it, shards of glass reflecting a sunbeam that shown for a brief moment only to get lost in the surroundings. One minute, they were there; the next, gone.

In my humble opinion, there's nothing worse than to look and hope for something, and discover that the thing for which you were looking and hoping was either a falsehood or no longer existed. This nightmare affirmed that feeling.

• • •

IN THE dream, Michael and I were back in school, walking on campus, heading to our Kali martial arts class. He'd been dating Linda for a time now, and had nearly decided to stop taking the course because of his girlfriend's dislike for violence. I was trying to convince him otherwise.

Sam, the trusted, eccentric bookstore owner I went to for support, for some unexplainable reason (well, it was a dream) ran unstably on his bad leg behind us, arms flailing, dreads waving wildly in the wind, yelling things I couldn't decipher.

And John and Alex and Linda debated mindlessly a few feet behind Sam, covering inarguable topics that would only arise in an aimless squabble on the street.

STATUS

The walk seemed to go on forever, and in this chaotic scene with nothing to latch onto, I repeatedly attempted to persuade my friend as the brick walkway plastered in students and surrounded by trees continued and continued and continued.

A group of dark clouds hovered, and rain started lightly only to worsen, until it pelted our skin with a frightening ferocity.

Honestly, with my memory distancing itself like it was, that I recalled this much was a feat. Regardless of the circumstance, I always expected to hear the assuring statement for which Michael was known: "Back to the good life." At the tip of my brain, I knew it had the word "life" in it, but struggled to remember the rest. When he didn't say it, the scene went black, and all I heard was silence…

• • •

SWEATY HAIR fell over my forehead and into my eyes as I sat up and forward in bed. My heart raced, and I breathed almost as deeply as when I seized, nearly heaving.

I couldn't remember my best friend's most notorious proclamation! This was a significant loss, and—though it went against logic—I wanted to reach out for it and plead for it to stay, as if it was something tangible. And yet I just sat there, and looked at the mess I'd made of my bed covers.

How much longer could I take this? The distress over losing what grounded me? Anti-anxiety pills would only help so much. Sure, I could pray that God would allow me to retain my memories, but I approached prayer differently than most. I didn't believe in requesting circumstances that made life easier. Unless, of course,

He willed it. In which case, upon requesting His will, He'd show me mercy in His own timing.

But anyway, I kind of felt it was time to accept this was beyond my control. Only then would I be able to start living and make new memories.

• • •

PART TWO

17
SEIZURE OVER DINNER

THE WOMAN looked as horrified as I felt. She handled the seizure well initially, as it began like the rest. But she lost her composure when it moved into other unfamiliar areas of the brain, and evolved differently than any I'd experienced in my thirty years of having Epilepsy.

I was at the fast food joint Wendy's, perhaps a couple hundred feet from my home, for dinner. The food was far better there than McDonalds behind it, but the management, employee cooperation, and speed at which they completed food orders were severely lacking.

JOSHUA HOLMES

After, let's say, twenty minutes of standing in line, waiting for my 4 for 4 meal, I finally was able to take my full tray back to a tiny two-person table.

Computer bag on the floor at my feet, I had my visual aura, purposely lay my head on my arms, and then blanked out for a few minutes. Harmless enough, right? I bumped my tray with a few leftover fries and a brimming, large Frosty, but it didn't tip and I hadn't scared anyone yet; that I knew of, anyway.

Her youngest son pointed at me when I arose from my seat, the bag at my feet tipped, and I stumbled closer to his booth.

"I'm having a seizure," I said. "Help me." I imagine I looked like a wanderer in bad weather, searching for cover.

"Look mommy, I think he needs help."

In my dream state, I had imagined that one, specific child was the person who would end the seizure. Some might call it a premonition. I didn't know what to term it, but it was definitely ironic.

I stumbled closer, and pointed at the second boy with her. "He's the one supposed to help me. Not him." I had no idea why I said such a thing.

Terror filled her eyes, her maternal instincts on high alert, but I said it again, still beyond rational thought.

Another man got up, moved closer to me, and offered to call an ambulance.

"Please no," I said. "I'm having a seizure."

"Ok son," the man said. "I won't call."

"That boy there," I said. "He was the one supposed to help me!"

STATUS

The woman's eyes grew even larger; so fear stricken I sat back down. Even in my stupor, I didn't want to come off as a crazed threat, neither to her and her family, nor to the other diners.

I was weary, but at the same time, was driven by a piercing headache, and a strange urgency to leave before the Police and EMTs determined the comfort or discomfort of my evening.

"I'm sorry," I said to everyone, picking up my computer bag by its strap. "I'm leaving now."

"Are you sure?" asked the man. "Isn't that risky?" Anyone recognize that question?

I suppose it probably wasn't the safest choice, but I am one of the most stubborn people you'll meet. He couldn't have kept me from leaving the premises, not at that point.

I walked over to him, placed my untouched Frosty before him, and said, "Just drink this for me. I didn't touch it."

And I walked unsteadily out of the Wendy's side door, into the darkness, across the street, to my apartment.

• • •

18
DISTANCE

THE LAST meeting opened the door to probably the most interactive exchange in recent church history. Nearly all of the verbal members had contributed, and the rest had listened, or so it seemed.

JOSHUA HOLMES

And yet I felt a distance between the couples, perhaps an alienating distrust. I couldn't say for sure, but it was as if the expressed positions were too casual for the others in the room, or they weren't believable enough. Scorn and skepticism appeared to cross everyone's face at one time or another. All around the circle, I sensed a suspicion that ebbed and flowed.

From the beginning, I assumed the age difference within the group was an influential factor, causing what might be referred to as a 'generational divide', a leeriness that hindered any relationship growth.

For all I knew, they were afraid my seizures would disrupt their unity. I know it was a fear of mine. It wouldn't be the first or last time it crossed my mind.

You could argue that I got it all wrong, that it was a matter of misperception (as the politicians on TV regularly claimed), or that I was just super sensitive, attribute it to any number of other shortcomings, really. I perceived a sincerity in their previous attempts at encouragement, after all. But I was still learning the ropes of life group, and as I'd always told those closest to me, "I'm no good at playing the guessing game."

• • •

I THINK MORE than anything, I struggled with the fact there were some things about the group that rubbed me the wrong way, and yet week in and week out, I showed out of some moral obligation, or to abide by a set principle. But I couldn't pinpoint the real reason.

The truth of the matter was: If you didn't commit to the process, you wouldn't experience the meeting the way you were

ELECTRIC

meant to—with a newfound degree of joy or mourning at the growth or loss of another.

I was committed, no matter, and that evening—despite my struggle—something interesting occurred. Foster Monroe, the frequently absent, tired truck driver, returned. He even went so far as to talk, and, specifically, to me.

With a stretch and a yawn, Foster said, "It's Chris, right?"

I looked at him, offered my hand for a shake, and said, "Yep. Nice to see you."

"Thanks, he said, returning a firm shake.

"You too."

"Anything good on the job front?" I said.

"Trucking companies in need of drivers?"

"No. Unfortunately," he said. "Lot's of time on my hands, actually. And not on the road."

I went ahead and explained how I could relate, as my freelance work was time-consuming and currently consistent, but had come sporadically in the past.

"But you make up your own schedule, right?" said Foster. "Being freelance and all…"

"I do, yes."

"Well, how would you feel about exchanging numbers?" said Foster. "So we could have lunch on a slow day?"

"Sure," I said. "Sounds like a plan."

Like most meeting nights, I quickly left with Hank, eager to escape the serious tone and pending interview questions, and to get home, far away from tradition. Only tonight, I had a new contact number in my pocket.

I especially enjoyed the return trip, because I got to probe Hank about his real opinions, not only about the lesson, but also regarding the actions of Foster Monroe. Whether it yielded substantial responses was something entirely different. And yet it accommodated the tug of war inside me.

• • •

19
TAKING STEPS

HAD IT really come to this? Taking steps to prove I was serious about dating someone I thought I'd known very well, but instead only knew enough to conclude she was a player?

I mean, I realized she had the right to date whomever she pleased, but at least she could've started with one, and if she really had to, moved onto another in time. But to overlap dates, and give two separate men false impressions? I just never presumed she was that type. Who was having a good laugh at my expense now?

Or was I totally off base? Imagining worst-case scenario when I ought to be imagining the opposite? Was this Mary Grace's way of weeding out the wrong guy? Was she closely monitoring each response to decide which suitor would be the beneficiary?

If I could settle on one thing, it was this: The internal debate had to stop. The back and forth was for the uncertain. I wouldn't project confidence if I were in doubt.

STATUS

• • •

I STARTED WITH the most basic of steps: A rose dozen purchase and delivery from the one and only Royer's Flower Shop.

The business had thrived in York, PA as long as any I could recall, that all-glass structure always full of flowers and plants to gift someone special.

"Twelve white roses, please," I said at the front register. "The best for the best." I was all about corny at this point. Whatever won Mary Grace back.

There was a number of bloomed Hosta hanging in planters overhead, some petunias and tulips at my feet. Just steps away, an employee watered the remaining floral selection.

"And your note?" asked the florist. "You want it to say what?"

"For my angel, Mary Grace," I said. "Love Chris." The florist repeated it back to me, to be sure he wrote it correctly. I nodded when he was done, but having witnessed all that I had, I struggled to approve of my own words.

I handed over the absurd amount the florist demanded of me. *All I know*, I thought. *Is she better like them*. I suspected Mary Grace's response to this gift would indicate how receptive she would be to any future steps.

• • •

JOSHUA HOLMES

20
REPLACEMENT

INSTEAD OF mourning the disappearance of my memory, subconsciously clinging to what was, I preferred the notion of accepting the past, pushing forward, and replacing the hurt by creating new memories. If, for whatever reason, images crept up on me, I would do my best to neither re-live things, nor to wish for a different outcome. I would refuse to dwell, and would rather look ahead to the future.

Of course, it was only natural—during the transition process—to try and make sense of what did pop up, to rationalize the irrational. And everyone operated differently while living through the process, perceiving and handling things in their own individual way. I was no exception.

Michael and his seemingly constant presence had arisen fast, been there for a time, and then diminished just as speedily. His face and words didn't come back as much, but his past existence and most hurtful act of rejection occasionally revealed itself. I consciously decided to forget him, but it was funny how the psyche dealt with loss.

• • •

THERE WERE a few partial reminders—scratched photos in broken frames and a disintegrating drawing in blue—of and by Michael in my room that hit me especially hard before bed one night. They were tucked in behind my massive stack of books, just

ELECTRIC

about hidden but not quite. How they had gotten down there, and why I hadn't tossed them sooner was beyond me.

The irony of it all was that I'd looked in their direction numerous times, passing them repeatedly, distinctly picking up nearby novels just beneath the closest electric socket. And yet, this night they landed in my sightline, and it dawned on me that—even as my recall ability declined—they were probably responsible for my choppy reflections and nightmares.

Bottom line, I couldn't have anything out in the open that might hold me back, physically, psychologically, or emotionally. Nothing that would disturb me or stir up my condition.

So, former best friend or not, I put away Michael and his pictures on the rear shelf of my deep hallway closet, where he and his vestiges could no longer deter me.

• • •

21
EASIER TO SEE

THE BLUE lens glasses were a shield for me, yes, and transformed my world's overall hue, yes, and altered my seizure types (still unsure if for the better), yes, and lengthened my days, yes, but—looking back—they also made it easier to see what exactly was the root cause for a lone seizure, or, alternately, for a cluster of seizures.

Before the glasses, the seizures could have been pinned on any number of different causes: Stress, lights, or excess stimuli in any form. There might have been a couple different responsible triggers, but it wouldn't have been out of the ordinary to blame multiple, co-existing triggers. Not now.

One of the first things I did, upon returning home from my bizarre seizure at Wendy's the other night, hidden by a bent yet functional glass frame, was to check my medicine container, to see if I'd forgotten my Keppra XR. Not until this aesthetic change had I been so severely and quickly affected by a dosage miss. Never had it been so clearly noticeable.

And, immediately, in my tiny bathroom, on my sink, I saw that, in fact, there was an untouched, full amount in my morning dispenser. I shook my head in disgust. I knew forgetting happened, but it just really annoyed me. Every time. Even so, I knew ahead of time I could anticipate a long night of hard Grand Mals, and had an explanation. How's that for finding positivity in a bleak situation?

• • •

DUE TO the rough night I had as a result of missing my medication, I had to temporarily put aside Nadine's project, and all things job-related and technological.

To date, Nadine's novel was edited, compiled, and published, her ebook was created and available for sale, and a small following had been established. It was a start that, once my med levels were again therapeutic, I would build upon.

Not to frighten anyone, here, but I didn't want to go into Status after assuring her it could and would never happen. In my late twenties, I might have continued staring at my computer, to assemble her

STATUS

book's marketing campaign, at my own expense. And still, I would've felt guilty for not achieving everything. But, you know, I'd matured. It could wait.

And hadn't Nadine encouraged me to relax, after all? Told me that life was too short to stress? Hadn't I told her I'd do my best? I remembered that much, for sure. And, regardless of my previous concern over deadlines, I was presently in total agreement with my client.

• • •

22
PROACTIVITY

JUST AS I had taken the proactive approach to win back Mary Grace, I decided—in order to defeat my perception of distance within the life group—to approach the members in a similar, proactive manner, a method I'd failed to enact just yet, and one I hoped would encourage greater interpersonal connection.

Would it work with Mary Grace? At this point, I could confidently shrug my shoulders. Would it work with Lanny, Leah, Ham, Sylvia, and Foster? Again, I could confidently say, "It's impossible to predict." Although, I surmised the life group members would give me a better sense when the meeting started here, and sooner rather than later.

I started with Lanny Galt, assuming he'd be most inclined to oblige me with an engaging anecdote or ironic work tale.

"Hey Lanny," I said. "Heard any new yarns at the office lately?"

JOSHUA HOLMES

Hank appeared to shiver when I initiated the talk, as if scared my boldness would come back to haunt us both.

My question caught Lanny off-guard, and his response was delayed, but he tugged at his suit coat collar, and gladly entered the spotlight, his temporary, serious expression immediately replaced by a wide grin. "As a matter of fact, Chris," he said. "I heard a good one today."

Leah Galt grinned and said, "If it's the one I heard earlier, I can vouch it was pretty good. Not an anecdote, per se. But a humorous joke."

"Why don't they play poker in the jungle?" said

Lanny, jumping right into it. No one knew, so after a brief pause he said, "You give up?"

Everyone laughed, and said in unison, "We give up!"

"There are too many cheetahs!"

I rolled my eyes and snorted. "Pretty good, Lanny. Pretty good." At this, Hank also shuddered.

The joke, however, even rose above Ham Reed's sadness, as he let loose an authentic chuckle in between Kleenex blows and nose sniffles.

Sylvia Fanning still lifted her chin and said, "Hum," but then, afterwards, for the first time in my experience, she smiled.

Foster didn't have much to add, but—between the glisten on his skin, and rare burst of energy—you could tell he appreciated Lanny's effort.

I turned to Hank. "You get it?"

ELECTRIC

"Sure," said Hank, offering a slight, nervous grin, but nothing more.

I knew I hadn't done a lot, but I had taken action. I went out on a limb and started a comfortable, low-key conversation each one of us in the life group seemed to appreciate. I still didn't yet fully trust my own judgment since miscalculating Mary Grace's cues, and yet I somehow felt closer to the couples before me, not nearly as detached.

The new feeling of intimacy convinced me the risk—at least within this unit—worked, and was worth the reward. But the risk didn't stop here.

• • •

23
PRESSURE COOKER

I WASN'T THE best at expressing just how I felt, even when I was in a pressure cooker. But I still planned to go the extra mile to let Mary Grace know the feelings with which I was dealing, especially as they related to her.

I was praying that one of these steps would do the trick, because I didn't know how many new ideas I could come up with. I didn't doubt my ability to foster my existing ideas, but how many different ways would I have to approach this to convince her I was the original she wanted?

One resurfacing pattern you'll notice as I move forward is my constant return to my innate talent—fine art—when it's imperative that I emote. Sometimes, writing helped. Usually though, stress and frustration led me back to the drawing board. This time, it was the need for control over *something*. *Anything*.

Unlike my place on Waters Road, across from the bowling alley, as opposed to a sheet-covered, chalk-smeared floor, I worked instead at a spacious table that accommodated an easel and fabric piece, reclining in a comfy chair on wheels. I kept the TV on low in the background, and started a portrait of my crush.

I initially had that same sickened response when I deeply considered I was doing a portrait of someone who'd so obviously moved on without me, but persisted in spite of it because I knew this reaction would lead to a favorable depiction.

I started sketching and blocking it all in. My focus became so honed in, I got lost in the process, and before I knew it, all that negative energy was gone, channeled directly into the lines and shapes that comprised the portrait.

Hours would pass, and her portrait went through numerous stages. I had a decent likeness that turned into an exact replica that turned into an abstract and cycled all the way back to a duplicate image. I didn't even worry about the back and forth, rise and descent and rise. It was part of the journey.

Some might find my commitment to such a task a bit extreme—possibly even strange—but I approached my drawings like a professional. I'd come to learn that 80 hours would yield me a piece to be proud of. All else aside, I expected 80 hours would yield a piece Mary Grace would be proud of, and perhaps cajole her thoughts back where they ought to be: On me!

• • •

STATUS

24
TIMESLOT

NEEDLESS TO say, I had been disturbed—even haunted—by my dissipating memory, and spent my nights trying to recall entire bygone events with Michael, assessing my emotions along the way. That is, until the fragmented nightmare, until I chose to let go, and started spending my evening hours differently.

I couldn't say that it was an immediate, short term fix; couldn't say it would be a permanent, long-term fix, either. Only God could offer these promises. But I could say the choice was an adjustment.

Nevertheless, I used that allocated timeslot I previously wasted to reminisce, instead as a block to calm down, to settle so I didn't attempt sleep wired over something beyond my control.

I still relaxed in my bed, propped up on my pillows, legs tucked under the covers, lamp on in the corner, some nights the mounted TV playing on low, other nights pure silence ruling as I flipped through a good book.

I started to see that—the more I utilized the timeslot for things other than reflection, whether it was for prayer, reading, talking, or watching TV (in that order would probably be best)—my mind didn't automatically grasp for the story pieces that recounted my history with Michael. And I didn't feel the need to seek them out, in all their scattered glory.

• • •

25
PART OF ME

WAS THERE a psychological element to these blue lens glasses, after all? I know I compared them to the VNS device, and initially decided they differed.

But I asked this question because some time had passed, and the longer I used them, the more they felt a part of me. I also felt this, years ago, when the VNS device was inside me, under my clavicle. Sometimes, you looked in the mirror at your reflection, and couldn't help but think about the treatments on/in your person. I was fairly certain anybody with a VNS or pacemaker install would back me up on that.

The glasses started out feeling foreign (because, well, technically, they were) but then—through repeated use—I normalized them, people associated them with me, and the accessory instead felt regular and necessary.

I supposed you could say the same about my anti-seizure drugs, but I'd never had the same feeling. And, likely, because I consumed the one, and wore the other.

Despite all the changes I faced, and despite their ongoing nature, they weren't anything to which I couldn't learn to adapt. As I continued to live, to go out in public and to group, and I didn't seize where I had before, the comments lessened, the strange looks decreased, and the worry wasn't so prevalent.

• • •

ELECTRIC

NADINE HADN'T said anything about the seizures or glasses in quite a while. Neither issue had been detrimental to her book release date or her marketing strategy. I'd adapted to the job, and hadn't given my client any recent reason to worry.

I could have told her about my cluster, however, in my view, there came a time when you kept things to yourself. I didn't see the point in sharing more about my physical struggles, especially since I was again therapeutic, and she'd been good about trusting me despite her concerns over Status.

Following a restful work break and an additional day off after my seizure-filled night, I jumped right back into her marketing strategy. And we had a good talk about steps we'd have to take to press onward.

"For each online marketing outlet," I confidently said. "We'll need your photo, a nice quality, welcoming image."

"Oh ok," said Nadine, pulling on her brown-blond streaked hair. "I think I have one or two. Anything else?"

"As a matter of fact," I said with a smile, glad to offer direction. "We'll need a nice bio write-up. In other words, what do you want your reader to know about you?"

"I see," said Nadine, an evident, building excitement on her face. "I'll have to think about that. But I'll try to have something to you soon."

"Wonderful," I said. "This is good."

"Anything else?" *Slow down, Nadine.*

"Actually Nadine," I said, still pointing the meeting where it needed to go. "We have a few other things to do, but we don't want to take on too much at once. Let's get these two things squared away, and then we can address the rest."

• • •

26
A BIT RISKIER

DISCUSSION TIME had felt unnatural to me from the start. Good lesson or not. I doubt anyone missed that early comment of mine. I realized it was a sincere, albeit blunt and possibly alienating statement, but—when all was said and done—it was a part of transition and integration, no matter what setting we were talking about.

Everyone settled in at his or her own pace. It just so happened I didn't immediately transition or integrate into the life group, and braced the open forum even more slowly.

Now that I spoke to the reality of transition and integration, I'd like to remind you that—during our last meeting—I boldly attempted to soften the overall tone, to unite everybody.

I had waited until after the lesson to seek and initiate an anecdote or good joke, waited for "snack time." And as I already noted, the risk was effective, as walls seemed to fall.

That said, I knew I would only experience more gratifying results if I participated with the other couples during the lessons. I could add my two cents, I just found it a bit riskier, and, frankly, didn't want to offend anybody. No matter, I would say a few words tonight.

• • •

STATUS

THE LESSON of the week—like all weeks—was basically a synopsis of the material the pastor covered behind the pulpit over the weekend, and was comprised of a series of questions that, I assumed, was meant to incite an engrossing group exchange.

"The reading is out of the first gospel," said Lanny Galt. "Do we have any volunteer readers?"

"Going over Jesus's final days," said Leah Galt. "The betrayal and abandonment before His Death and Resurrection, of course."

I put up my arm, and announced, "I can read it." Hank handed me his Bible to reference, since I'd accidentally left mine at home.

"Thank you," said Lanny. "Nice to have you contribute."

Perhaps the group would appreciate my offer. If they didn't already, perhaps they'd take me more seriously.

I went ahead and read like one or two chapters in Matthew, and everyone nodded their heads, contented.

Ham Reed was bawling by the time I finished. "I still can't fathom how He dealt with the betrayal!"

"Nice reading," said Foster, surprisingly without a yawn. "You captured it well." Hank, per his usual response, quietly agreed.

Sylvia Fanning, as expected, nodded and hummed.

Again the switch up in member participation led to a more exciting debate over the text, and, generally, to a nicer time. I didn't want to take credit for the evening's success, however my second risk (and I still considered it so) did help.

• • •

JOSHUA HOLMES

27
BOMBARDED

MY THOUGHT was this: If I bombarded Mary Grace with reminders of us, they would force her to reflect on our past relationship and stray from Mr. Perfect.

As far as I was concerned, as long as I put Mr. Perfect in questionable territory, I still had a chance. As long as he didn't achieve that relationship plateau, where he might be considered a permanent fixture, my reminders were bombarding her perfectly.

It wasn't like the reminders were traumatizing ones, either. They were prompts that should have jogged good thoughts about me, perhaps stronger thoughts of us together.

She'd already taken her time, though; had already been careful to keep me hanging in suspense and deep in uncertainty. I was having auras, left and right. Had a Grand Mal over it, too. Granted, I might have been uncharacteristically suspicious, but she easily could have put that to rest and instead chose not to.

I found it kind of ironic, also, that I—having recently decided to release the clipped, unfinished dreams that tormented me—was trying to re-instill old images and events into someone else's memory bank.

So far I'd sent flowers (spent money), and composed a portrait (spent time), both things thus far failing to encourage the response I wanted: A guaranteed, guilt-ridden return. I wished I could have gifted them under different circumstances, too. But as the saying went, "It was what it was." For my second-to-last attempt at con-

ELECTRIC

vincing her to come back to me, I decided to utilize my other talents in design to make a typographic visual just too hard to ignore (spent creativity).

A colorful, web banner, otherwise known as a .png file, I figured, with a corny yet cute message, or an invitation to return to me, all done up in serif and san serif font combos might do the trick. I again was grasping at straws, nearing the bottom of a dry well of ideas. And yet, if I beautified an impactful note as only I could, and posted this to her email, or even to her numerous social media accounts, perhaps it would have its desired effect.

I noticed how frequently I added the word 'perhaps' to my considerations. To be frank, I couldn't afford to have my efforts lead to anything preceded by hypotheticals. I wanted nothing but successful reunification. Right?

• • •

28
TIMESLOT REFINED

FOSTER MONROE'S compliment during life group filled my head as I was winding down before bed later that week. I considered it, and felt it was a good thing to remember and thank God for before falling asleep.

But it didn't stop there. I thought about the times he had attended, how he'd been silent for the most part, and, specifically, how—after a notable absence—he'd spoken to me (of all people) and posed the possibility of getting together for lunch or dinner.

I had successfully refined this timeslot so that my memory issues wouldn't overwhelm me. And taking the step had turned the block into a wonderful and often relaxed, healing period.

Why couldn't I set aside a different timeslot for Foster and me? Not only just to eat up, but also so that any erroneous thoughts or images couldn't creep back into places where I didn't want them. So we would create new, positive memories there, and outweigh the otherwise broken, detrimental ones. Why not take full advantage of the more-than-obvious opportunity presented me?

I turned over onto my side, leaning upon my elbow, and reached for my cell phone, which was plugged in and charging nearby on the mattress. It was a little late to make a call, but if I didn't try now, I'd struggle later. I pulled the phone closer, and dialed Foster Monroe's number.

• • •

29
AMBIGUITY

WHEN I was blessed with seizure droughts, it was especially easy for me to credit the blue lens glasses, and when my Epilepsy slammed me, it was just as easy for me to doubt them. From my vantage point, it appeared the same thing applied to my friends and family, as they would praise my glasses in the good times, only to question them in the off times.

I don't recall this happening with each new change in anti-convulsant. Perhaps once or twice when I experienced and mentioned

STATUS

a Grand Mal drought. I hadn't changed my medicine line up in several years, and supposed prescription changes weren't as apparent as those attributed to my blue lens glasses.

I knew it all went back to uncertainty, to disbelief. Epilepsy, alone, was frightening to the informed and uninformed. Add blue lens glasses to the picture, and it just enhanced the ambiguity. On top of that, I'd endured so long, and accomplished so much (and I say that proudly and humbly), people didn't grasp what I went through behind closed doors, and the incredible difference the accessory made in my day-to-day life. I bet you Nadine would second that.

• • •

THE PHOTO and bio write up Nadine and I agreed upon complimented one another pretty well. I had to increase the image resolution a tad, and convince her that—if I were in her shoes—I'd consider and replace some select wording. Two things I seemed to do with all my clients. But other than that, we'd managed to finish the steps I suggested, and we were set to take on a couple more.

"Now that those two things are up," I said, right after submitting the material to each retailer's technical services. "We can add a few other things, if you like."

"Chris," said Nadine. "If you think I need to add to this, then I trust you."

I always loved when we got to this point. It made things so much simpler when the client put his or her faith in my recommendations.

"Well yes," I said. "I think connecting an rss feed to your blog, a Google channel, and including additional links to your home website, portfolio, etc. would serve you well."

"How can I help?"

Another way to see whether rapport had been established was to watch the client's desire level to assist in any capacity.

"There's not a whole lot here," I said. "But you could email me a list of links you want your reader to have access to."

"I can do that, I think."

"I'm sure you can. All I need from you now," I said. "Is permission to add these things."

"Permission granted."

• • •

30
FOOD

As a reminder to the group that I was making an effort to be inclusive, I committed to bringing a couple food items to the next outdoor pool party. No big dishes, but food items nonetheless. Yes, I knew that, as an invited attendee, it was the socially appropriate thing to do. At the same time, I guess I just hoped they appreciated the act, and expressed it somehow, as it was something new for me.

We were in a cobblestone farmhouse, somewhere in Red Lion, a small place where I hadn't yet spent any time. By all appearances, it looked like it had been around forever, water-stained ceilings, crooked floors, and chipped paint just a few indicators.

ELECTRIC

Hank didn't get to tell me whose place we were meeting at, but—through the process of elimination—I excluded all homeowners in the group, except for Ham Reed.

From an olive, fabric couch, Leah Galt passed a list around. "On the left, you'll see your names," she said. "On the right, the tentative food and snacks."

"I'll be manning the smoker," said Lanny Galt, in the same ancient couch. "Chicken and ribs with my specialty marinate."

"And if anyone here hasn't had his marinate," said Leah. "You are in for a treat!"

"I'll get some chips and dip," said Ham, in better spirits than I thought was possible. *Is it the mention of food? Or that we are at his home?*

On the lone, tan fabric recliner, Sylvia Fanning used her left index finger to scan the paper, seemed to raise her chin after perusing each food item, but managed to save her hum for the moment she wrote her name next to her snack of choice.

"Foster Monroe called me. Told me he'd bring the flavored drinks," said Leah. "I suggested soda and tea."

Hank and I were on the floor, sitting Indian-style before an unmatched coffee table draped in lace. We were the last to receive the list. Like we were last during Q&A time. Not sure why we so often landed in that order, but it gave us time to decide on our area of contribution.

"I can pick up some pretzels and cookies," I said, glad the options were still available, adding my initials to the list.

Hank laid claim to water and crackers.

I felt my commitment got me a few extra congratulatory nods, perhaps an additional smile.

I had hoped for some feedback, at first, and again I think the group was warming up to me.

• • •

31
FRUIT BASKET

So I know that I said I couldn't afford hypotheticals and that reunification was priority (and it had been the case), but until Mary Grace gave me some kind of take on my shower of gifts, I was still caught in the same limited position: Seeking to achieve her approval via present giving.

Unfortunately, I knew she was under no obligation to speak her mind or to show me any sign. She didn't have to tell me why she thought how she thought, why she behaved the way she behaved, or what might convince her to reconsider us as an item.

Familiar with my own personality, with what made me tick, however, I knew deep down I would only keep this cycle going so long. Propose a gift, and wait for a response. And then I'd push aside my desires, and turn to logic and reason. In other words, I'd consider other available options.

It seemed I'd said this a few times now, but it felt I had exhausted all options nonetheless. Even so, I decided to invest my energy into another winning outlet. I'd watched a funny sitcom—*Everybody Loves Raymond*, in fact—once on the strengths and weaknesses of fruit baskets, how a year supply of them could be nice to have around, but equally overwhelming if not eaten in a timely manner. Among the characters, havoc ensued and appreciation for the item quickly turned to disdain.

I probably should have taken the hint. The basket was hardly creative, and the trouble topic in the show, but all those apples, pears, and bananas wrapped in cellophane? I hoped a duplicate gifting would remind Mary Grace my intentions were pure, I was thinking of her, and that I was still trying to impress. At this point, with nothing to gauge her feelings, with no way of knowing what else Mr. Perfect had done, I was willing to try this and any other avenue (even more spent money).

And yet, as much as I hated to go there, it would be my final stab at victory before I started to seriously consider the walk away. Remember, the first, hard yet worthwhile walk I had to take before approaching the dreaded second? The one that helped me depart with my head held high? I absolutely loathed defeat, but failure was a part of life, and—as any experienced senior would wisely affirm—I wasn't able to omit that part from the process.

• • •

32
ENOUGH

THE ANTICIPATION for my dinner with Foster Monroe, believe it or not, was enough to refute my memory woes. I had hoped the meeting itself would also help in this way—and I still thought it could—but I didn't foresee the benefit of the wait that preceded the dinner. I was truly grateful for the added bonus.

I had been right the other night. It had been a bit late for the call to Foster, but he'd been gracious. I thanked him for his compliment at life group, told him that it had been on my mind, that it reminded me of our previous conversation, and—by the time our discussion came to a close—we'd agreed on a day, time, and place for the first get-together.

His kindness outside the life group context impressed me, negating any disturbing images. And, as I said, to enjoy feeling eager was so nice; the early excitement was unexpected yet welcomed.

• • •

THE FIRST meeting with Foster was reminiscent of my first night of bowling league with Stone, in that it was demanding, nerve-wracking, intriguing, and exciting all at once. It only differed in that the latter included physical competition.

Considering he was unemployed, and I was making just enough to get by, we chose to eat at the grocery store, Weis Markets. The same place I walked to and where I worked on my design projects everyday.

"I went ahead and bought a couple pizza slices," said Foster as I entered through the automatic doors and glanced at the place where he sat, under the bright, white lights at one of many round, wooden tables. "Hope you don't mind."

ELECTRIC

"Not at all," I said, stopping beside Foster, greeting him with a shoulder pat. "I'm gonna go put in an order for half a rotisserie chicken."

"So this is where you design then?" he said, taking in all the beer aisles, floor displays, and neon signs on the walls. It was a far cry from Penn State's food court at the HUB, and the Art Institute of York-PA's nonexistent one.

"Yep," I said with a smile, sitting there, still waiting on my meal in a bag. "And consult with clients. Can't forget that."

"Definitely not," he said with a smirk. "A unique setting, for sure."

"It works for me," I said. "Smells yeasty at times, but 'unconventional' is the name of the game! A different setup never hurt anybody."

"True."

"Thing is," I said. "I like what I do. And how I do it."

"Yeah. Me too," said Foster. "Probably why it makes being out of work even harder."

"My thoughts, exactly," I said. "But I'm confident a new opportunity for you is around the corner."

"You'd think there just has to be, wouldn't you?"

A kind, Weis employee was nice enough to bring the chicken to me.

"You think you could ever work daily over here?" I asked, lightening the mood with a minor topic shift, a wad of chicken in my mouth. "Or is the front seat of a truck and a highway the only place for you?"

Foster paused. He looked down at his empty plate, and then back up at me. "You know, I didn't stop and think about that until I was out of work. But I think you hit the nail on the head."

"Hey," I said, picking up our mess and nodding at the exit. "You ready to go?"

"Sure."

For two guys who didn't normally say a lot, unless otherwise prompted, Foster and I managed to have a good conversation that was comfortable. I wasn't usually quick at anything, but I knew immediately this had been fun, a good decision, and I would do it again.

• • •

33
CURIOUS

I WAS CURIOUS to know if some of my questions about seizure changes due to blue lens glasses would be answered with an additional glass coating.

With what we already knew about Zeiss—that cobalt was the hue that improved things—whenever I had an aura, I wondered if three dunks would make a difference for me. Would four or five dunks, for that matter, closer match the Z1 F133 color, and soak up more of my trigger?

When Dr. Dune dunked my lenses once, and then twice, there was a noticeable difference between the two. The second was so much better. It was exciting, and, without exaggerating, changed my life.

As I prepared to meet with Nadine, to go over the retail sites' layouts, and basically conclude this part of the design/publishing/consulting process, I thought about what was next. I'd continue as

STATUS

a design consultant, no doubt. As for my glasses, I did want to experiment. An increase in color application couldn't harm me. In fact, it could only help.

• • •

"JUST A heads up," I said. "From here on out, all I can do to change the look of a retail site is bother the techies."

Nadine looked at me half amused, half perplexed. "What do you mean?"

I laughed. "In other words," I said. "We both submitted the core marketing components, and added your blog and links. We have a general idea of the layouts, but how the techies build it into their websites is up to them."

"And you can call them to inquire about adjustments, but not much more?"

"Well," I said. "My hands aren't totally tied. With a lot of practice, I've learned the process."

"The process?"

"You know, how to get around the service reps to the designers who know what they're talking about," I said. "It's nothing complicated, just tedious."

"Then I'll leave it to you."

"All I'm saying is that our approach from here on out will be different."

Nadine shrugged. "That's fine."

We turned to my laptop screen again at my dining table with the embracing zebras, where I had all her customized author pages pulled up.

"That said," I continued. "After giving you cause for concern, there isn't anything to be nervous about. I think you are going to love what they've done. I took a look before you got here."

There were some minor aesthetic things I'd alter if it were mine, like always, but it was preferential.

This was my client's call. And if she was satisfied, so was I.

She clapped her hands again, and looked to the ceiling. "I'm so excited!"

A minute later, she took a thorough look at them all, saw every step we took amounted to what I'd described, that her personal photo, bio, and book were all there. Her face just lit up.

We discussed sales, how she'd collect her earnings, how she'd have to set up her bank accounts. It was probably the most concerning part for all my clients.

She also gladly paid me another nice sum of money. That made me smile.

"Any other questions?" I said. "Or are we good for now?"

I knew that particular question usually didn't yield anything in the moment, as it put my clients on the spot. I also knew, however, that she'd have a question or two before long. My clients always thought of something on their drives home.

"I'm very pleased," said Nadine. "I think we're good for now."

• • •

ELECTRIC

34
STORY

I'D PARTICIPATED to the best of my ability in life group. I'd also embraced my feelings of disconnect and discomfort, and observed positive changes following my personal attempts to improve them.

It didn't occur to me, though, until I ran out of ideas to show my desire for inclusivity, how many times I had evaded the interview questions, so I didn't have to share the specifics of my life story. And also how my deflections had to influence the group's perception of me.

"There's not much to tell." That had been my original response that seemed to allay further probing. Now that I was aiming for more, now that they'd all shown me some warmth, I felt it was time to give them a taste of my life story. I know I was thinking ideally, but perhaps it would change the way we currently interacted. Just maybe it would help Ham defeat his sadness. Or encourage Foster to talk. Or for that matter, push Sylvia to say something in addition to her hum. Or present Lanny another platform to spread his joy, and Leah another opportunity to serve as a support.

• • •

MY WORDS were limited in number and information. But I did say a piece here and there, and the group must have picked up a little about me, and naturally drew conclusions.

I believe I had told them when I was saved, and when I was baptized, and where I'd gone to school. I hadn't talked much about work.

JOSHUA HOLMES

And as I predicted, the group had more questions for me. Not necessarily ones presented in the same order or asked verbatim, but direct, info-gathering questions. This time, though, I didn't resist.

I learned in counseling school that—used properly—self-disclosure could be a good tool to foster trust. In my internship with Dr. Webber, and later, in my design work with the pastor and Nadine (to name just a few examples), it led to closer relationships, too. Exactly what I wanted here.

I took the opportunity to explain my Epilepsy diagnosis, how the group could—at any time—have to deal with it, my botched brain surgery and subsequent physical losses: in my eyesight and sensation, my recent experiments with blue lens glasses, and generally tried to explain how it made meetings like these difficult for me. At the same time, I clarified my desire to be an accepted, contributing member.

When they all responded in their own unique ways—crying, sweating, laughing, agreeing, and humming—but together they accepted me, and my story to boot, it changed everything. In a way, I wished I'd done it sooner, because I felt the mutual trust that had been missing, and a new freedom to speak without hesitation.

• • •

PART THREE

35
POSTICTAL STUPOR

IT TOOK more time than anticipated to get all the glass and dried blood from my skull. In my usual Postictal stupor, I lay there, scraped up and heaving, obsessing, clawing at the broken remnants and darkening crust. It didn't help that I twice connected, headfirst, with the brick and concrete in a populated area while waiting my turn to get my hair cut.

My stylist (who wouldn't get to me today) worked perhaps twenty feet away, at the Hair Cuttery. A dental office, Wine and Spirits, Adam's Jewelers, Nittany Pizza, Sweet Frog, and GNC squeezed the place. And pretty tightly, like most strip malls.

JOSHUA HOLMES

Nearly all the parents and children stepped around me as if I were a gas slick that could dirty their shoes, but, thankfully, one woman stayed with me, sitting by my side in the chilly evening air.

"My name's Greta," she said. "Everything is going to be fine. I'm here." She rubbed my sweaty bangs from my forehead, and repeatedly assured me. Her voice was as smooth as butter.

The story, I'd hear again and again, went as follows: As the seizure spread, moving from aura to generalized, I lost my speech yet made some guttural noises, I twisted backwards like I usually did, ricocheted off a brick column that supported Queensgate Plaza's low overhang, and fell directly onto her, knocking her over and hitting my head the second time in the process.

Of course, I felt badly about it. Wished I had a semblance of control over what my body did. But if it had to happen this way, I was glad I'd landed on Greta, a sweet, shapely, auburn-haired girl who immediately made me forget Mary Grace, attracting me even in recovery.

She gently brought my hand from my head and to her lap. "You keep picking at that, we'll have a mess. Help is on the way."

"Help," I fearfully said. "I can't."

"What do you mean you can't?" said Greta. "We need to take care of your head."

"Please," I said. "No EMTs. I'll be fine."

• • •

AND I would be fine. But not before first dealing with the Emergency Medical Technicians. Granted, Greta was a big help. In fact,

ELECTRIC

I can guarantee she picked up where I left off. I wasn't much help for the majority of the time they were there, disorientation overwhelming me because I was so exhausted. I was able to make clear, however, that I didn't want to go to the hospital. As was always the case, I didn't want to get caught in a wasted evening, and later with absurd medical bills.

The EMTs looked to be a pair of rookies on test run. Couldn't tell if they were from Yoe, or from White Rose. The ambulance was feet away, ready to transport. But I wasn't.

Greta explained to them how she'd come to be involved, told them a few of the demographic things I must have told her, although I don't remember anything I spoke while in my haze.

I felt my face. "My glasses," I said. "Where are they?"

"Here Chris," said Greta. "Right here."

She opened her purse, retrieved them, and handed them to me. They were badly scratched, but I put them on right away.

"Please let them look at your head," said Greta. "You hit it twice." Negotiation with me in Postictal wouldn't work.

"They'll charge me!" I said, shaking my head no. "They say they won't, but you get a massive bill a week later!"

In the past they'd made a mess for me to clean up, an unnecessary debt I had to spend hours on the phone convincing my insurance company to cover.

They tried to negotiate a while longer, and finally realized—logical or not—I'd continue to argue against a ride to the York Hospital ER.

"Just sign here, then," said EMT rookie #1, at last. "And here." I objected again, but eventually consented.

JOSHUA HOLMES

"And you're sure?" said EMT rookie #2. "You knocked your head pretty good."

"Yeah. I'll walk home," I said, pointing. "Thanks. But I live just back there."

• • •

I WAS SURPRISED Greta stayed, after my objections and upon hearing how close I lived. In the past thirty some odd years of seizing, on occasion, random nice people waited and helped, but then usually left once things settled. Greta, on the other hand, went above and beyond, and in many ways, reminded me of the type of woman I wanted, sensitive and committed even when it wasn't required.

"Can I drive you home?" asked Greta. "Help out with anything? Remember, I'm not an EMT."

"You don't have to," I said. "But I'd appreciate it."

Even in my stupor, in my mind's eye I could see my old bowling teammates, Burke and Bender, celebrating the offer, urging me to say yes.

"No really," she said, concern still on her face. "It would make me feel better."

"In that case," I said. "I'll take you up on your offer."

As much as I'd love to tell you our first encounter was this dreamy, intellectually and physically stimulating experience, it wasn't. I managed to direct her to my place, and—wobbly on my feet—she helped walk me inside to my apartment, where she sat on the couch and waited for me to wash my head clean in the bathroom sink.

STATUS

When I was finished, I remembered to get her a drink from the fridge. My speech was still a bit slurred from the Grand Mal, so I was hardly conversational. We kind of just sat there together in silence, until she said, "You need rest, hon. And I need to get going."

I wanted her to stay more than you know, but I also agreed with her. She was right. I must have looked as exhausted as I felt. And even though she was gorgeous, I saw the fatigue in her eyes.

Still gimpy, I got up and opened the door for her.

"Thank you so much, Greta."

"My number is on your coffee table," she said.

"Call me when you're feeling better."

Romantic? Hardly. But it was how she first entered my life.

• • •

36
EMAIL

I DIDN'T MAKE it to life group after the seizure. My head wasn't bloodied anymore, but I was still cut up and in a lot of pain. The ache traveled from my skull, and down into my neck and shoulders—areas I previously injured during a Grand Mal, mind you, and had worked tirelessly for five months last year to rehabilitate. The thought of going through that again was disheartening, but I wasn't going to make any early assumptions.

More often than not, I still would go out—whether it was to bowling league, a movie, or life group—even if I felt badly. If feeling trashy were the determining factor, I wouldn't ever do anything!

When I didn't go out, that's how you knew I was beat. I had hit my threshold. Needless to say, I was hurting enough.

I called Hank, told him I wasn't able to go, and he was kind enough to honor my request to tell everybody why. He also asked for prayer, which was evidenced by a sympathetic email from the group, promising thoughts and prayers.

I wasn't surprised, per se, that my life group took the time to encourage one of their members who was currently experiencing physical discomfort. I'd been at the meetings when they asked us all to remember other struggling people in prayer.

While I struggled to connect with the group, at first, they'd always been nice. In fact, thinking on it, the Galts gave me little paper notes with seasonal sentiments around the holidays.

Excluding the weekly reminders about the upcoming meeting location, however, this was the first, full-length online note via email, written specifically to me for encouragement purposes. I enjoyed it, and thought it was pretty cool.

I liked to think my commitment to the group—regardless of the involved difficulty—was starting to pay off.

• • •

37
LAST TIME

MARY GRACE'S silence bothered me at first, no doubt about it. But with each dollar spent, and exertion of creative energy, with

ELECTRIC

each hour passed, new gift sent, and no hint of appreciation, or sign that I was doing anything right or wrong, it grew easier to let go.

I was, no question, shocked and confused that she hadn't taken a moment to contact me, through any means, at any time during my pursuit efforts. Not even to leave a phone message, to either tell me I was sweet and it meant something, or that I had no shot whatsoever.

The only things that made sense were that Mr. Perfect had changed her as a person, and he was possibly dictating the ordeal. Or maybe Mary Grace thought—with continued silence—I'd eventually put two and two together. Or, most cynically but realistically, perhaps she wasn't even the woman I'd always thought she was and seen her as. I'd experienced that in my lifetime, too.

I sort of wondered how this would impact future visits to the neurologist, if she would be just as evasive, and if things would be awkward during the check ups, but that aside, nothing else crossed my mind.

In any case, I had tried wooing Mary Grace for the last time. I was done. No regrets. To fall back on a well-used cliché: Why cry over spilled milk? Am I right?

Everyday she was easier to release, too, because—more and more all the time—my mind was drifting back to an even sweeter, kinder, more thoughtful, more attractive woman named Greta.

Which reminded me…I was feeling better, and I owed her a call.

• • •

JOSHUA HOLMES

38
JUST SO HAPPENED

"So YOU had an incident over here at Queensgate Plaza, huh?" said Foster Monroe. "Heard about it the other night."

I hadn't told anybody in my network where or when I had the seizure, just that I had, in fact, experienced one, and needed to stay in.

"Where'd you hear that?" I asked, kind of perplexed. "I didn't even tell Hank."

We both sat at the round table we used last time. It smelled especially yeasty in the Weis beer café today.

"It's a funny thing, actually," said Foster, hardly the same quiet guy from before. "Not the seizure. But how I heard about it."

"Funny how?" There was nothing like a dinner story to refill my memory bank.

"So I drove over to a local temp agency to see if a rep could help me find work," he said. "You know, at this point, I'm open to anything."

"Right," I said, leading him. "And you heard it there?"

"So I walk in and the job rep looks exhausted. She introduces herself, invites me to sit, apologizes to me for her appearance."

"Uhuh."

"She says it just so happens she literally, moments before, got in from helping a guy who had a bad seizure over here. I knew you had Epilepsy, and you worked close by. I connected the dots."

"She could've been talking about anybody."

STATUS

"Yeah, I suppose," said Foster. "But you told me you are a regular at the strip mall, like almost everyday, right? I just assumed it was you. And then I heard it again at life group."

"The rep," I said. "Was her name Greta?"

• • •

39
TIME BEING

DR. DUNE was more than accommodating, thank God. Upon hearing of my bad seizure and the resulting scratches on my blue lens glasses, he immediately understood the situation's gravity, and gave me a time to come into his office.

"So let's take a look here," he said. "You say they're pretty beat up, huh?"

I handed over the case containing the damaged goods. I temporarily wore a backup. "Yeah. I'm really not the type to exaggerate."

The office was empty, so there weren't any inane distractions. In our fast-moving world, I always enjoyed when things came to a temporary stand still.

Especially if the halt would improve the customer service, which appeared to be the case.

"Yes," he said, laughing after lifting the pair with his skinny fingers, and examining the marred glass. "I'd say you need a fix."

He stood up and, towering over me, found my file, to see about my insurance. It would give us both an idea about what exactly were my options.

JOSHUA HOLMES

It opened the door for me to discuss lens color experimentation, and the possibility of a third or fourth application of blue hue.

• • •

"I WAS THINKING," I said, looking at all the plastic frames hanging on the walls, at every name brand you could imagine. "About something the other night."

"Not too hard, I hope."

"Never too hard," I said. If only. "But, seriously, I was thinking about my blue lenses. I really believe a darker blue lens would help me."

"Oh yeah?"

"And I only say so now, since I need to replace the scratched ones."

Wearing backups, light hit me in excess from all sides, and I quietly hoped he'd continue to understand.

And as if on cue, he said, "I understand."

"Well, for the time being two dunks was a game changer. It affected how strong my auras were. Not to mention numerous other things for the better, and some things I'm still trying to figure."

"So you explained earlier," said Dr. Dune. "And it really is fascinating, I must say."

"A third dunk could soak up even more light," I said. "Which could make an even bigger difference! I was hoping you'd be willing to do it for me."

"Well, of course I can do that," said Dr. Dune. "But I'll have to get new lenses, more blue tint, and set up the tint machine."

ELECTRIC

"Thank you. I realize I'm requesting a lot, but I need them like ASAP," I said. "Since I'm using a spare pair without any color. I'm very exposed."

• • •

So NADINE didn't call immediately following her ride home, but not long after that. I'd venture to say about an hour after I finished with Dr. Dune. I was right, however, that she thought about something in the car. Everything was good, but a minor concern crossed her mind. I wasn't surprised. New things always came up.

"Hi Chris," said Nadine. "I realized, heading back to my place, that a couple book covers weren't centered."

"Yeah," I said. "It tends to happen a lot."

Her observation of the layout glitch now meant the project wasn't finished.

"How hard would it be to make them all look the same?"

Requests like these always evoked mixed emotions for me. It meant more work, which was good. But it also meant my clients weren't yet fully contented, and they wouldn't be without a resolution, which was worrisome. That—in addition to feeling exposed—was a loaded combination.

"I can bother the techies for you," I said. "Have them retry centering the images."

"Oh right," she said with a laugh. "Forgot about them."

"Like everything else," I said. "It'll take time. Possibly days. Possibly weeks."

• • •

JOSHUA HOLMES

40
RELAXED

THE DESIGN project might stretch for days or weeks, I didn't know, but life group was set to start on time, as it routinely did.

Hank arrived at my place especially early, because, he explained, the get-together would unfold differently this night. He didn't want to miss anything.

He also said the group finished with the lesson study guide we had referenced during the gospel discussion, and, in my absence, they had agreed to a movie night. *In other words*, I thought. *They all want to relax.*

I missed the last meeting, yes, but I desperately needed time to heal. Feeling much better about my physical condition, about the state of the group, and about my membership, however, I was ready to return, and, I don't know, watch with the group a clean film I hadn't previously seen.

The way I'd felt about life group in the beginning, I never foresaw experiencing any degree of relaxation. And yet, here I was in the dark, on a plush couch, feeling connected and at peace.

The movie was called Risen, one of the year's many Christian depictions of Jesus's life, death, and resurrection. It seemed they had told the story from every imaginable angle. This picture played out through a Roman's eyes.

In any event, the Galts promised accuracy and pretty good acting. I appreciated the film; had nothing bad to say about it. But I was more intrigued by how I was feeling, or not feeling (depending how you looked at it), in the current setting.

Lanny and Leah were, no doubt, proud to present their movie, and sat together with giddy expressions on their faces, akin to expecting parents looking forward to a host of congratulations. Leah would occasionally whisper, "Oh, I like this part!"

Again reflecting on abandonment, Ham was crying. He knew the story well, and still took it in as if he'd never heard or seen it before. I didn't think I'd witnessed such sensitivity in my life.

Throughout the film, Sylvia hummed. I still thought the lone iteration was incredibly slight, yet—I had to admit—her response fit the context of each scene.

I assumed Hank enjoyed the flick. I think we all would, unless he said otherwise. And I really didn't expect he would express a dislike for it. I figured if he were asked whether he liked it, he'd say, "Sure."

What a crew, I thought, amazed every time by the group make up, yet at ease. Made for quite a ride.

• • •

41
RETURN CALL

"**H**EY THERE, Chris," said Greta. "You must be feeling better." *Aah. To hear that buttery smooth voice again. So nice.*

A lot had happened in the past several days, and this phone call was much needed. This time around, I didn't struggle with nerves, or have any of those pre-contact butterflies in my stomach. More experienced now, I instead felt excited.

"I do feel better," I said. "Thank you."

"Wonderful," she said. "That's so good to hear."

What I found refreshing was the fact she genuinely did sound happy to hear the news. There was no doubting the authenticity.

"The question is…" I said. "Are you recovered? I know they, the seizures, can be tough to see."

"I am fine," said Greta. "Don't even think twice about it." I said ok, but that was like telling an on-duty cop to forget a runaway thief.

"So you're in job placement," I said, jumping topic. "Very interesting." And it was. I'd studied it in graduate school, and—though I rarely discussed it—had briefly worked in a similar position.

"I never told you that," Greta said with a laugh. "Chris, have you been doing a background check on me?"

"You better watch out," I said. "I'm full of surprises."

"Is that right?"

"Yes indeed," I said, continuing the playful banter. "When I'm not designing, I'm investigating."

We laughed together on the phone. It was fun to joke with someone I was attracted to.

"But, truthfully," I continued. "As if our mutual experience weren't crazy enough, I had another with one of my friends, and, ironically, I think one of your clients."

I went on to convey the story Foster had narrated for me, as close as you could duplicate a "he said, she said" account, and we

ELECTRIC

spent the next forty-five minutes talking and laughing about the irony of it all.

"I'm shaking my head here," said Greta. "You are friends with Mr. Monroe."

"I have to admit," I said. "It almost sounded too coincidental to be true, at first. And I did question Foster. But once I was convinced, once I accepted the plausibility, I was eager to tell you about it, and to get your reaction. I thought it would make for some pretty entertaining conversation!"

• • •

42
SYNONYMOUS

I HAD SO many new people in my life, synonymously saying and doing positive things to, for, and with me, an array of fresh experiences to think upon, that the disappearing memories and incomplete dreams about Michael grew even scarcer.

The scarcity, as you will recall, was what originally bothered me the most. Almost to the point of obsession. But now I was so occupied, many times so busy—between work, life group, and Greta—that I didn't have the time or energy to dwell on the missing pieces.

My eyes were heavy, and I momentarily closed my lids as I pulled back my bed covers. I was surprised I made it this far, as some nights—in full dress and under bright lights—I hit the sack and fell asleep on top of my comforter, blue lens glasses and all.

The thing of it was: Like a refrigerator just filled to brimming after a shopping spree, my memory bank was now chock-full again, overflowing with new enjoyable events I remembered specifically and completely, and that made it seem as if missing memories of Michael were never an issue at all.

Instead of spending a whole hour in bed strategizing over how to better utilize my time, relying on self-imposed yet effective distractions (not that these actions were inherently bad or anything), I was embracing the mattress earlier, having my nightly talk with God, and then immediately falling asleep.

Which would likely happen this night. I did manage to sequentially take my meds, turn on my fan and sound machine, turn off my lamp, pray, and then settle in. That fun-filled conversation with Greta would be a comforting exchange to visualize as I drifted off.

• • •

43
GOOD THING

ALL AROUND, my curiosity about and eventual acquisition of darker blue lens glasses was a good thing.

My trip to Dr. Dune's office was not a wasted one, as he did a wonderful job replacing my scratched lenses, adding color to a new set, and subsequently returning them without excess delay.

I gladly put away my back up pair of glasses, no longer felt overly exposed to the light, and gratefully relished the added protec-

STATUS

tion. Negating more of the stimuli; Talk about minimizing a needless life stressor.

My seizures hadn't totally stopped (would they ever, really, if I thrived despite them?), but the third dunk of hue had significantly depleted my auras—to give you an idea, from roughly thirty a week, down to ten or less. The Grand Mals still occurred, but it seemed with even less frequency.

Cosmetics were never a huge deal for me, as I was far more concerned about function. Aesthetically speaking, though, I thought the updated pair looked better on me, that they were more masculine. In passing, people still stared at the color of my glasses, however it appeared to occur in a more positive light. For some reason, observers were torn over the paler blue, and were drawn to that which more closely matched the cobalt.

Like I said: Good things.

• • •

"It'll take time," said the customer service rep named Brenda, sounding more robotic than human. "Possibly days. Possibly weeks." You recognize that line? I prayed I relayed this same information to Nadine in a less automated tone.

"I understand," I said, expecting no different. "Would you please transfer me to the person above you?"

"I can, but they'll say the same."

"That's fine. Transfer me anyway. Thanks."

As was the case this far into a freelance ad campaign, I was back on the phone sifting through those who could and couldn't make the changes Nadine wanted.

It was taxing, yet still a good thing, since I was doing again what I had done multiple times before.

This exact scenario had played out more times than I could count.

"This is Charles. Tech Support Specialist. How can I help you?"

"Not sure if you can help, Charles," I said. "But maybe you can direct me or connect me to the person or group who can help me."

I was happy to reach the next tier, to explain what exactly were my client's grievances, and to emphasize that I was familiar with the timeframe script. I also was quick to add that I would appreciate a priority mark noted with the request write up.

"I will pass this along to the team," said Charles. "Can't give you a completion date, but I promise I'll move it along as quickly as I personally can."

"That's all I ask," I said. "Have a good one."

• • •

44
MEMORABLE

SOME OF the more memorable exchanges I'd hold close were those I experienced outside the immediate life group meeting location. In particular, when at church—the Sunday after the relaxing movie—several of the members went above and beyond to express

ELECTRIC

appreciation for my transparency and attendance, and in one case to remind me of an event upcoming.

To see that neither my early hesitancy, my appearance, my seizures, nor a 'generational divide' interfered was refreshing, and again gave me hope and peace.

Of course, the Galts were first. They weaved their way in and out of the narrow rows of bright pink pews immediately after the sermon, and came right up to Hank and me.

"Hank. Chris. You doing well this morning?"

"Yes. Thank you," I said. "You guys?"

"Oh we are good," Lanny said. "We just wanted to come over and tell you how nice it's been to see you come out of your shell. To speak up and show at group!"

"Just Wonderful!" chirped Leah, so excited, it seemed, she could fly circles around the sanctuary.

We all shook hands and wished each other a restful day, and as Hank and I were about to leave, Ham Reed pushed aside a cluster of attendees, and quickly approached us. *Wow,* I thought. *Aren't we popular today!*

Ham Reed usually waited for others to come and offer him consolation in one form or another, so it was already a new experience to see this side of him.

"I know I was emotional the other night, but I wanted to tell you that I enjoyed watching the movie with you guys," he said. "Wasn't it well done? Just what I needed to take my mind off work."

"Thanks Ham. I enjoyed watching it with you too," I said. "You're right. It was well done."

Ham shuffled on his feet. "Alright, well have a good week."

"Oh right, you too," I said. "Thanks."

Hank and I crossed the atrium while a recently created pathway still existed, and made it over to the coatrack, where windbreakers hung. Sylvia Fanning caught us as we put on our outerwear.

"Ah hum."

The sound was so isolated and unique, it had become oddly familiar. I knew it was Sylvia even as she stood in my blind spot.

"Hi Sylvia," I said. "How are you?"

"Good," she said, chin lifted. "Remember the pool party is coming up."

"Thanks. Will do."

She smiled and waved. "Hum."

Four meet and greets after a Sunday service. It was a marked improvement. I would remember the encounters.

• • •

45
EARLY YET RIGHT

I PROBABLY MADE an anxious decision. But still I couldn't say that it was detrimental. It was early, I admitted, but something about it just felt right. You know that feeling? The one you didn't even take a second to debate?

Having experienced the likes of Mary Grace, someone who did a three sixty in every possible way, I had since been careful to draw permanent conclusions about Greta. But again, that 'just right' feel-

STATUS

ing made it all the easier to anticipate learning more about Greta, to work at strengthening and sealing a connection. All it required was the proper setting, and I believed I had a good idea about that, too. Which ultimately led to the question that would prove either timely or untimely.

"Tell me if this is too soon," I said to Greta.

"But I have this pool party thing I was invited to.

There'll be food and drink and conversation with my life group members. Was wondering if you'd join me?"

• • •

"HONESTLY CHRIS, I would say, under normal circumstances," said Greta. "That it might be somewhat soon." Oh boy. Here it comes.

"I suppose it was hasty of me," I said. "But I felt good about it, you know?"

"And considering we learned a lot about each other right away... spent a lot of time together in person and on the phone... I can see why you would."

"If it's too early, Greta, I get it. I will go alone.

No pressure."

"No pressure here," said Greta. "Are you feeling pressured?"

"Hardly."

"And you're not retracting your invitation, Chris?"

I gulped; Got all flustered, which was what she wanted, I'd learn. "Of... Of course not, Greta. I'd love it if you would go with me. I guess I...I thought..."

"Chris. Listen to me." Pause. "First of all, I don't want you to get upset and have a seizure. And secondly, a pool party sounds fun!"

"Oh yeah?" I said. "So I can mark it on the calendar. A date?"

"Mark away, hon," said Greta. "It's a date."

I laughed, relieved. "I had to work for that one, didn't I?"

• • •

46
MIRACLE WORKER

"I'M TELLING you," said Foster. "That woman is a miracle worker." And more.

"I knew it the first time I laid eyes on her," I said. "Even coming out of a seizure."

Foster and I were meeting up for what, he warned me, would probably be the last dinner at Weis for a few weeks.

"Yeah," he said. "I'm like… I can't even think of the correct word… ecstatic right now."

"So Greta found you some work?" I said, downing another rotisserie at our regular table.

"And some good work?"

"Better than good," he said, nibbling on some pizza crust. "Great!"

"I take that to mean you got something in trucking."

"Can you believe it?" he said, crumbs spewing forth. "Exactly what I wanted! And in this economy?"

"I was hoping Greta would come through. But I just didn't know…"

ELECTRIC

All I knew, looking around, was that it appeared dimmer and smelled yeast-free today. I couldn't remember the last time the deli felt so fresh and the light so faint.

"She connected me to the right people, and set the ball rolling!"

I was glad to hear Greta pulled some strings for Foster, was proud of her and thrilled for him; Wasn't every day two special people in your life reaped rewards.

"I realize I said it before," I said. "But I had that feeling it was only a matter of time."

Our second discussion, I had been at a loss for words, and barely managed to give him the needed encouragement. I was glad I said it now.

"Oh, I know," said Foster. "And not to get all down in the mouth. But you know how it is. When you're going through the hard times…"

"Yeah," I said. "You don't always see things clearly. Or objectively, rather. Hard to put one foot in front of the other. Totally get it."

"So I start this upcoming week."

He went on to detail the likely route, the projected schedule, and pick up and drop off specifics.

"Wow man! That's awesome!"

"Like I said, I am jacked!"

• • •

47
DAY TO DAY

So AFTER exploring the ways I was impacted by the blue lens glasses, and exactly what I had to adjust to, the good, the bad, and the unidentifiable, the conclusion I arrived at was a familiar one: That while they helped, they were not an over night fix. You had to take it slow, day-to-day, and make changes when and where you could.

Speaking from experience, I (and my fellow friends with Epilepsy, I'm sure) had heard this mantra many times over, applied to each treatment plan, tested or untested, cheap or expensive, effective or ineffective, natural or medicinal. It was just another toss up, an experiment that aided some, and didn't others. But they wanted you to be a willing lab rat without any objections. How dare you express concern and demand concrete proof of positive results!

I had been fortunate enough, however, to come across that blog article with evidence; fortunate enough it encouraged all readers to consider the success of that young girl. I had been intrigued enough to test it out on my own. Dune played a key role, but, beyond that, there was no outside interference, no harm, no foul. And I had been blessed to see—in my personal life—more resulting benefits than setbacks.

• • •

REPORTING SUCCESSFUL fixes and completed projects was probably one of my favorite parts of the freelance process. And those, especially, that took days instead of weeks, because of my extra prodding on the phone. I suppose 'because of my honed communication skills' sounded better, but when was I ever politically correct?

"Nadine?" I said with zeal over the phone. "Chris here! I wanted to pass along some good news."

"I wasn't expecting to hear back from you so soon."

"Yeah," I said. "Well I wasn't expecting to call this soon, either. I spent a chunk of time finding the techies to resolve things. They gave me that noncommittal, timeframe answer."

"Maybe days. Maybe weeks," said Nadine with a snort. "That one?"

"Yeah. That one," I said. "But I took a glance at your site real quick this morning, and it looks like they made all the fixes."

"You're kidding!"

"No kidding," I said. "Just took speaking to the right guy, and some additional diplomacy."

• • •

48
PERSPECTIVE

I WOULDN'T ALLOW myself to lose perspective. And I prided myself on this, even if it first took analysis and critical thinking.

So I had experienced life group differently than ever before: feeling relaxed among the members. Didn't this uplifting change for the better imply a fairytale ending? The kind most readers expected?

Granted, they weren't an island vacation, a sit in the shade, kick off your flip-flops, and put your feet up on a wicker table set of instances. Yet with all my feelings of uncertainty, followed by my acts to earn approval, now in the past, that 'easier' meeting I wished for throughout emerged not only after I told my story, but even more visibly during movie night and at church.

Ideally, I would feel the same from here on out. Many other people would. But this wasn't how it typically fared in my case. It was never that easy for me, and that was okay.

That said, I wouldn't seal my demise by saying I couldn't feel equally adjusted, integrated, and at ease. I had grown a lot, and I supposed my chances had increased. I believe I said I'd watch the story play out on the first night, and, it was true, I had.

Now, nearing the end, I would say it again. Things would play out, regardless.

• • •

49
APPETIZERS

"I COMMITTED TO pretzels and cookies," I said to Greta, like an hour prior to the party. "The popular snack items on the list."

"The cheapest too," she said. "You think I didn't pick up on that?"

I smirked. "Purely coincidental."

"Nice try, hon. You do remember who you're talking to, don't you?"

I smirked again. "My memory hasn't been good, of late…"

ELECTRIC

She was driving us over to the Galts, but before we went that far, she told me she'd stop by a gas station, so I could run in and pick up the food.

"Although," I added, after a beat. "I never forgot who I was talking to. How could I?"

Managing the steering wheel didn't keep her from pulling into Exxon, and giving me a playful punch to the shoulder as I turned, unbuckled, and opened the door.

• • •

LAUGHTER AND discussion floated on the wind coming off the Galts' back porch. Not everyone had yet arrived, but it sounded like the early birds had already been ushered poolside, and were enjoying one another's company. Greta and I could hear it from the driveway, as we made our way beyond Ham and Sylvia's parked cars, through the grass, and to the party site.

Lanny and Leah had gone out of their ways to spruce up their back porch and yard, which looked as well-kept and grandiose as the interior of their home. The porch boards were freshly stained; the railing was adorned in white, Christmas lights; the lawn chairs were evenly placed; the nearby pool sparkled a crystalline blue. And the aroma of Lanny's special marinate covered it all.

At my side, gracing a red sundress, and matching red lipstick, Greta looked wonderful. Any previous comment I made about Mary Grace's appearance could be tossed. Especially the one stating, 'No one could beautify curves quite like her. Or genuinely present a grin that stirred something so strongly inside me.' Because in the moment, Greta's long, auburn hair, unique shape, and grin made any other aforementioned, strong feeling within a light tap in comparison.

We could see our elongated reflections in the water as we walked over to the center table. It already contained some of the food items on the list. I put the bags of pretzels and cookies down.

My date put her arm around mine, and as each interested life group member approached, I proudly introduced her. "Hello there," I said. "This is Greta."

• • •

EPILOGUE
ENDLESS PURSUIT

DAYS PASSED and the design projects were coming in consistently. Nadine and other former clients were returning, wanting my help. I was getting referrals in bulk. I was meeting new people outside work with greater ease. And fresh off Mary Grace's dismissal, and the introduction to and connection with Greta, I was feeling pretty darn good about things, excited about the present and the prospect of the unknown.

My social life had always been limited, as it was hard to connect with people who were frightened by my presence and condition, but—once I acknowledged the required, extra work—I began glimpsing hope at the end of the tunnel, and eagerly anticipating new developments. It gave me confidence and changed my outlook.

STATUS

As it stood, Hank, Foster, Stone, and I would continue hanging out and socializing the way we did—over meals, on the road, and during bowling league. We might even pursue some different activities. Who knew?

I was satisfied with how the whole life group scenario panned out. I chalked it up to a hard yet good learning experience. There were numerous other groups from which to choose, and, in time, I potentially could try them.

No longer tortured by my memory, I was working more hours, and—with my blue lens glasses—doing so responsibly. I was hitting my deadlines, updating clients, sustaining relationships, accomplishing personal goals, and, most importantly, chasing life's endless pursuit.

• • •

TRIGGER
A NOVELLA

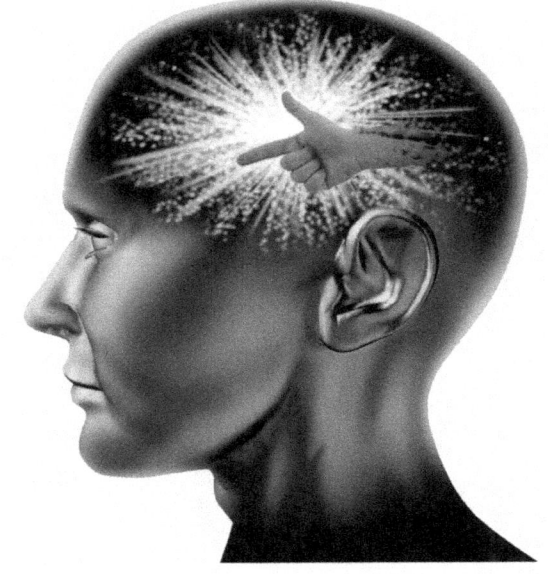

AUTHOR OF STATUS
JOSHUA HOLMES

PART ONE

PROLOGUE
OPEN CASE

"HELLO CHRIS?" said the high-pitched, Asian voice. "Is this Chris?"

"Who is this?" I said, more abruptly than I usually did. "What's this about?"

I'd been asked direct questions like this before. And mostly by evasive phishers. If the guy claimed he couldn't say because of security reasons, I'd know he was a telemarketer, and hang up on him.

"I'm calling with the Franklin County FBI field office." Franklin County FBI? Could it be legit?

My iPhone even verified this. A web search of the number further validated it.

JOSHUA HOLMES

What did that mean anymore, though? There'd been so much talk in the news about hacking and identity theft, Russian interference, propaganda, and so on.

Fear filled me, and my heart pounded in my chest. And as much as I know fear is senseless, I had been roused from a rare, deep sleep. I was forced into immediate thought, nearly convinced of a problem, definitely put on edge.

Hesitantly, I rolled over and sat up. *Focus, Chris!*

I was somewhat skeptical, but still very concerned.

Random rational and irrational possibilities began to consume me.

Was it tied to my year working as a clerk in the Clerk of Criminal Courts at the York County Courthouse? Did it involve one of the countless number of international housemates I'd had over the years?

"You must have called the wrong number," I said.

"There's an open case with your name on it."

So they had a case on me, but needed me to confirm my name. Huh.

"What do you mean an open case?"

If this was a ruse, they'd been very thorough about offering believable responses.

"A case," he said. "You mean my partner didn't call you about this already?"

"As I said, you've made a mistake."

"Please stay on the line and my direct superior will explain the details."

At this point, I was a nervous wreck, but quickly getting angry. I impatiently pulled at my covers. None of this felt right. Nevertheless, I stayed on the line.

ELECTRIC

The second voice that belonged to the "superior" was also Asian-sounding. I found this unusual, wondered how many Asians lived in northern PA, and worked in the regional FBI office.

My insides were quaking. My eyes were aflame in aural stimulation.

"Seriously sir," I said with more authority, anxious to get to the bottom of this. "Tell me what this is about."

I didn't know what can of worms I had opened. Was an FBI agent going to disclose a whole list of false charges over the phone?

I held my breath.

I SPENT THE next three months expecting every unidentified caller to claim FBI status and demand compliance. The Asian "superior" had hung up on me, offering no specifics, and my family and friends assured me afterwards that it was just a scam. But it didn't diminish the degree of trauma I experienced.

Granted, as a freelance graphic designer, I worked daily with many foreign customer service reps at the publishing houses. Some could be a pain, but many helped me take my design work to print stage.

That said, any time I had to deal with a telemarketer—regardless of ethnicity—I felt ill, and braced myself for a full-fledged seizure.

This, despite the fact I've never been in any kind of trouble, legal or otherwise. The mere plausibility of accidentally falling into mayhem promised turmoil.

I get it. To an extent, it sounds silly. Perhaps like paranoia. But it isn't. I knew my body well. All it took for a person with Epilepsy was one trigger. One prolonged stressor. One poke to my brain from that symbolic, pointing finger.

And when—around month four—yet another Asian voice sounded like an alert signal in my ear over the phone, I never had a chance.

"I... I can't talk to... uggh... to... you." I had been relaxing on the floor, putting a new filter in my sweeper, the TV on mute in the background.

"But this is Chris," said the Asian man. "Speaking."

His voice was so similar to the FBI copycat agents that I froze, assuming they'd returned to make my worst nightmares a reality.

There was no opportunity to brace myself this time around. The bag that was supposed to easily slide into my vacuum fell out of my hand.

"I'm... you... leave..."

"For your safety, sir."

A familiar lie that likely convinced the majority of the masses.

The guy didn't stretch the narrative like the other two, which would have been a positive under different circumstances. The brevity didn't exhaust the stimuli, however. If anything, the concision guaranteed my instant electrocution.

The filter rolled across the living room floor.

I started growling almost immediately. It was a new side effect. I couldn't intentionally speak, and yet I could hear myself make these absurd noises, short and labored as my head bounced off the hard vacuum hood.

The growling led to panting. And my panting quickly became more pronounced.

The vacuum handle tipped back; And then the whole thing fell over with a thud. The carpet dirtied in the process. The Asian man got an ear full of hot air.

TRIGGER

• • •

I
THE RETURN

I WAS ESPECIALLY defensive after the last concussion of 2016. It was justified, I still think, because it happened following my first Grand Mal seizure in four months.

Four long months. They had been unique and exciting months, because—after a nearly permanent hiatus wearing blue lens glasses—hope for an Epilepsy cure had found its way back into the picture. And then, instantaneously, the hope was dashed.

Not only did I have to quickly accept the seizure's re-emergence, but also, in time, the blue lens glasses' limitations, and the vexing injuries—temporary vision loss, distorted auditory sense, and a barrage of new, unfamiliar triggers (e.g. foreign telemarketers, for one)—to come.

"I'll get myself home," I said, stumbling towards the waiting bus. "Thank you very much."

The ambulance inched along next to me as I pushed ahead. Window down, the EMT leaned out. "If you have any other problems just give us a call."

On the surface, it sounded like a nice gesture. But they'd already repeated the instruction a million times. And I also knew they didn't care, that they were unkind.

One other lady and her kids—all of whom had originally helped me and were since gone—had witnessed the verbal abuse the medics earlier put me through, and could attest to my claim.

"How many times do I have to tell you?" I said.

JOSHUA HOLMES

"Leave me alone!"

For the second time in my life, my seizures had disappeared and returned. A little space to process and recover was all I asked.

"I've dealt with this guy before," said medic one. "Gave me trouble then, too."

I felt like I was listening to a pair of single parents grumble about a kid with an attitude.

"He's definitely stubborn," said medic two from the driver's side.

"Tough break," I said.

The EMTs moved at a snail's pace in their vehicle just parallel to me as I passed through a whistling wind and rounded the mall's walkway. Ultra Dental and Isaac's Deli were behind me. Hallmark and Giant were ahead.

"We can't just let you leave," whined the EMT. "We'd lose our jobs." *Would be one less headache for me*, I thought.

Concussed or not, I was determined to make my own choices, to escape those who stole my rights.

"I'll pay Red Rabbit a buck sixty before I pay you three hundred big ones for nothing."

Medic one tossed up his arms, chuckled, frustrated, as if that would dissuade me. He clearly didn't expect me to bolt after the Grand Mal. And he obviously didn't know my history—one, by the way, he and his crew had complicated.

"I swear you won't get charged anything!"

"If only that were true."

"I won't even document this!"

"Not if I can help it," I said. "I'm out of here."

ELECTRIC

"You can't."

"But I will."

Still disoriented, I picked up my pace. It was either now or never. What if my flight wasn't in my best interest? I guessed I would find out.

My blood pressure fiercely sounded in my ears as I climbed the bus stairs, paid my dues, and sat down in a daze.

• • •

TELEMARKETERS AND EMTs both were triggers, for sure. But so also were abusive clients. I didn't have many, but it only took one bad apple to spoil a batch.

Unlike Nadine—my last client and now a satisfied, published author and marketed success story—Adaline of The Festive Shore Deli & Foods personified the injustice that sometimes plagued the private sector.

She was a tallish brunette, brash at times, roughly in her fifties, and perhaps the most distracted lady I'd ever met.

Our introductory exchange was hardly impressive. I suppose it's possible my opportunity was blown right then. I was a referral trying to convince on a day the Internet was down and the design was undetermined.

I couldn't have seen it in the beginning, but when a friend later asked me if Adaline used the term "we" during our talks, that it was a good indicator of where her mind was, it dawned on me the conversations had been pretty one-sided.

JOSHUA HOLMES

"I have an upcoming meeting about the site," she always said. "I'll call you afterwards."

And, at first, I bought into it. She arranged meetings. But then the day of the consult arrived, and—surprise, surprise—something else came up.

"Can't meet today, Chris," she said. "A dog bit me."

Is this for real? I wondered. *A dog?*

And then after another re-schedule and some more time: "Hey Chris. Can't meet today. Was up all night. How about Monday?"

In my opinion, the excuses weren't very creative. And in both instances, I decided, I still would have attempted to keep my appointment.

Perhaps I was old school, but I considered the effort common courtesy. She could have just expressed disinterest in a re-brand and web design update, and given me a partial payment.

Instead, weeks without communication went by. My mind revisited every interaction, minimal though they were. Had something been said that changed her mind about upgrading?

To avoid further abuse—despite my severe exhaustion and mixed emotions about the dark day—I immediately returned to my project for the company.

On my couch, balancing the computer on my lap, I imagined she and her "team" were watching the site develop from their end. Like my reciprocal clients, I expected she would call with change requests.

The pastor who had met with me, asked me to design a children's book a couple years ago now, and pulled out last minute offered me my first taste of professional rejection. And it burned, no doubt.

TRIGGER

Little did I know that Adaline would repeatedly offer similar tastes, and the few empty exchanges I'd had with her would just be the start.

• • •

2
ANOTHER START

ONE IMPORTANT person in my life—my short, thick friend of few words, Hank—started the next night at my apartment by affirming his agreement to pursue a new social activity.

I pressed the issue of seeking the martial arts after I'd exhausted my passion for bowling, and realized a more physically demanding commitment would accommodate my client-related angst.

My bad seizure experience during league, and my history of studying Kali, Jiu Jitsu, and Tae Kwon Do also fed my desire to seek a different avenue.

Some selfish reasons there, I know. But I also wanted Hank to spread his horizons. I figured he just needed some encouragement. And while Hank probably would have continued at the alley, he eventually consented.

"I'm willing to try it out," he said, scooping a bite of Talenti gelato. "Haven't done it before, but I'm willing."

Intently listening, I ran my hand through my brownish hair, and stroked my goatee, which was starting to curl wildly.

JOSHUA HOLMES

I had been a loner so long that it was nice to jump into different activities with another person (e.g. bowling, life group, and now karate). That we were friends made it easier and better.

I should also add that our regular hangouts at my place were quite enjoyable. We no longer attended the same church (as I moved on to a nondenominational), so it was the perfect time to catch up with one another. And, to an extent, it picked up where our growth group left off. Better yet, we didn't have to abide by any unspoken morés.

"You know you can decline," I said. "Just speak up."

"I know," he said. "But yeah, I think I'm up for it."

"Awesome," I said with a nod, also downing a Talenti gelato container of my own. "We won the bowling tournament in our first season playing together, after all. Nothing left to prove there, right?"

We both looked at the trophy on my bureau. Hank had his award back home. "Uh yeah," he said. "Right."

I smiled and reached out to him, offering my hand to complete our secret handshake.

Our first night, Hank and I braved heavy traffic, and arrived at the York Shotokan Club dojo thirty minutes late. The place was rather isolated, perhaps a few miles off the highway, and was somewhat hidden on an elevated, grassy tract of land.

Hard to recall, I briefly thought back to the day I trekked off campus, across North Atherton Street, and sought out training in graduate school with Michael. The venture was different yet similar in some ways, and the same in one regard, as a nervous excitement filled me en-route.

ELECTRIC

Thrilled and curious, we presently located two open seats on an old, fabric couch pushed against the wall, and minded our own business as we sat down. A few parents and children occupying the rows of chairs just ahead looked in our direction and then away.

The evening would serve as a transitional sort, one of observation and preparation.

The students had already lined up, stretched, and moved into practicing the various Shotokan stances, kicks, and punches. They were consistently spread out, filling the well-kept gym to capacity.

One major difference I noticed and to which I'd have to grow accustomed was the way they introduced the style. There was no specific sequence; They jumped from move to move, combination to combination, kata to kata—a strong test of muscle memory.

"Doesn't look like we'll be doing anything tonight."

"No."

I had spoken on the phone to Sensei before we drove out here. Through the receiver, he didn't sound as eccentric as the ponytailed teacher in State College. He'd invited us to watch, promised a further discussion, and to help us if it was the right fit, so I was expecting his entrance any minute.

"But if we can pay our fees and get our gis," I said to Hank. "Then we will have accomplished what we needed to."

"True."

"We'd be set to start on the first of the month. Right on schedule."

"True."

As I suspected, Sensei eventually came out, introduced himself, and summoned us to his back office.

JOSHUA HOLMES

He was a tall man with a calm demeanor, a low voice, and piercing blue eyes. Direct and to the point, he put us through a pretty substantial interview.

There was an application to complete and submit. Like the interviews of the growth groups, our answers to the questions gave Sensei a general idea of our personal and professional backgrounds, and proved we posed no danger to the youngsters in the class.

It went about as smoothly as it could have gone.

• • •

3
BY MY SIDE FOR NOW

I STILL TRIED to do lunch at the Weis Market Beer Café (now offering wine, by the way) with Foster Monroe when he was home from a truck run, but he was always on the road. Came home perhaps once a month.

More often, however, as was typical when you landed a girlfriend, I found myself regularly dining with Greta. And having a fine time doing so.

I liked to think I was pretty easily contented, and this small tradition of meeting at Greta's employer, TempStar, and leaving together to eat out proved it. Formal companionship and tasty nourishment was more than enough for me.

I hadn't dated many girls, and none so wonderful as Greta. I wanted our relationship to continue.

TRIGGER

And, to guarantee this, I was well aware I needed to go the extra mile to please her. Change routine every now and again. Add interest. Introduce a twist to absolve any potential doubt about us.

It went against my nature, but I said to Greta around noon on a Monday, "How would you like to try something different today?"

She looked at me with surprise. "You losing your zeal for store food?"

"I don't know," I said. "Just want to keep the outings fresh for you is all."

"Oh how sweet," she said, tipping her head. "Very thoughtful."

I smiled. "I did think it through."

"You always have been a thinker."

"This was just one of my better thoughts."

"I would have to agree."

"Well? What do you say?"

"Switching things up is a good idea," she said. "I'm all about fresh. But we don't have to, you know."

Did that mean it was about time I threw a curveball? Was that the hint?

"You're right," I said. "We don't have to. I just figured…"

"You figured," she repeated.

"I did…"

She turned towards me and placed an index finger over my lips. "I'm excited to test the waters with you. Let's try it another day, though," she said. "Seriously."

But was she serious? I thought.

"So, my lady," I said after a beat, placing my hand on the small of her back. "Our usual then?"

Greta nodded. "Salad at Weis sounds good today, actually."

JOSHUA HOLMES

It seemed she hadn't yet tired of our regular lunches. So I said, "To Weis it is."

THE LARGE, round tables had been removed, and a number of booths had been installed. The soda and ice machines had been pushed over and shelves holding large wine bottles lined the open wall.

"Good day so far?" I said, sliding over in the seat.

"Appeared as though you had a number of files on your desk."

"I guess I had quite a few," said Greta. "But it is a good thing. And, so far, it has been a lovely day."

"I know my day just got substantially better," I said with a smirk, placing my hand over one of hers.

I genuinely meant it. Greta had stayed by my side through the close of life group, through my memory issues, through the struggles with my blue lens glasses, through the transition into new activities, but, most significantly, after witnessing numerous seizures in public, which gave me hope for us.

"Is that right, Chris?" she said. "How's that?"

"Yeah," I teased. "You see, I've been eating lunch with this cute girl. She's really something."

I continued to find her physically attractive, especially the curves and long, auburn hair, and loved to have her at my side whenever possible. I enjoyed her presence, and never tired of our random conversations.

The issue had never been finding a girl who liked me and appreciated my company. Instead, it was about locating that one female

ELECTRIC

substantial and intelligent enough to understand and look past my triggers and subsequent shaking spells.

We looked at each other and smiled.

And then the conversation took an unexpected turn, the light tone leaning more somber.

"I did want to run something by you…"

"Okay," I said. "Sure."

"You have had a lot on your mind of late," she said, matter-of-factly. "Anything you'd like to tell me?"

I snorted. "You don't miss a thing, do you?"

She was right, but I didn't think it was a good time to discuss my insecurities.

"And you are a master at evading probes," she quipped.

"It's nothing, really," I said. "Between the seizures, work, and starting karate, I've been preoccupied, yes."

I still found it hard to believe we'd come together following Mary Grace's insensitivity and one of my episodes at the Queensgate Plaza, and closer still days after, when I boldly called the number she'd given me the day she dropped me off at my place. And yet we just seemed to gel.

She picked at her salad and wiped her mouth. "I see. Well I think there's more to it."

Most recently, she had listened to me voice my disappointment over the Grand Mal return and my confusion about the various triggers. Unlike many, she was sensitive and assuring about my situation. But for how long would she empathize?

JOSHUA HOLMES

Michael and Linda had expressed embarrassment over my condition years before and dispersed. Mary Grace had gone on a date with me, only to drop me on a dime without explanation for Mr. Perfect. And, frankly, with my past significant others leaving me behind like they had, I just didn't know whether the kindest woman in my life would remain.

So she'd heard some things; Not everything, but enough to peak her curiosity.

"We have plenty of time to get into details later," I said. "I promise I'll share my thoughts, but for now, let's just enjoy our last few minutes together."

In truth, I would probably stall. Greta's possible exit plagued me like a head cold.

• • •

4
CARDS

IF I played my cards right, I could stall a while longer with Greta, perhaps, but I couldn't delay my six-month appointment that afternoon at Wellspan Neurology, which normally meant I would struggle to avoid an encounter with my former crush, Mary Grace.

Her actions still relatively fresh, I just wished I could get this over with, see my doctor, inform her of the seizure return, update records, and leave without crossing additional paths and stirring trigger-inducing emotions.

TRIGGER

And for an hour, in a hard seat at the edge of the segmented waiting room, I managed to elude contact with anyone. I got lost in thought—putting myself at risk, really—first returning to my initial attraction to Mary Grace, watching her from the stage on graduation day, and then to that awful day I happened upon her with another man. Mere hours after our date, she and Mr. Perfect were making out at his red sports car just outside.

And I very nearly went on to relive my successful efforts to divert that love fest in the parking lot, the good part. But I didn't get to. I was rudely interrupted.

"THREE TIMES, Chris!" said Rhys, my current Physician's Office Clinical Assistant (POCA), a shapely blue-haired, twenty two year-old girl. "Three! Be glad the doc didn't cancel your appointment!"

"Oh, I'm so sorry," I said, getting up and following after her through the automatic double doors. "I must have drifted off."

"I'd say so," said Rhys. "And I bet I know about whom, too."

"I bet you do."

A young mother, Rhys mentioned her child every now and again, and had no problem scolding her patients in much the same way she would a testy infant.

"Just so you know, Chris, Mary Grace is very busy today. You shouldn't concern yourself about running into her."

After stepping out of my shoes, I got on the scale, winced at the number. "I suppose you're right. But you know how she is. Looming large over the office and all. You can't really blame me."

JOSHUA HOLMES

When Mary Grace rounded a corner, even busy, her domineering omni-presence brought to mind a lioness guarding her cubs in a rugged savanna, or the number of adolescent minorities who used to loiter outside the West Manchester Regal Theatre, claiming a spot on the curb that clearly wasn't theirs. An obvious violation, if there ever was one.

"You're funny, Chris." said Rhys, filling out a chart and leading me into a barren room. "The doc will be in momentarily."

I could see into the hallway from my perch. I supposed Mary Grace had just as much right as me to traipse around the office.

Which meant she could interact with whomever she wished, including me. What if that hypothetical interaction grew hostile? What if the hostile exchange led to a bad seizure? Surely, I couldn't rely on her for help any longer. Every possibility my brain could create emerged in the silence. With each passing moment, however, it appeared we might
miss each other.

As long as she didn't interfere with my treatment.

• • •

5
WEATHERED

I WAS DISAPPOINTED about the seizure return, because I started to believe my sentence was up. I had allowed myself to imagine a future without the condition, a life absent of so many disruptions, one less suffocated by others' fear.

ELECTRIC

People could deny their fear all they wanted, could downplay it after the fact. But I heard and observed the horror in their voices and faces, and felt the disconnect when I returned to the place where I previously seized.

And yet, as had always been my motto, "It was what it was," and I had to keep going, to roll with the punches. I allowed myself to contemplate the hurt, but then continued seeking my pursuits.

Now in my late thirties, I'd weathered nearly every trauma in every location, and understood the necessity of pushing on when you didn't think you could anymore. It required more, physically and mentally, but I felt I'd achieved a new plateau where I placed less importance on suffering.

That's not to say I didn't have my moments of suffering, as we all do, or that I didn't ever over-react, since I occasionally lost my cool.

But I had 15 years of collegiate life to learn to adjust, and about four years of freelance design work to alter my approach to Epilepsy and its surprises. And I saw positive change, which is always a plus.

Granted, I addressed general illness at the first sign of its presence. But I didn't see any weakness in trying to catch a sickness before it took root.

The main thing I had to watch for, as I've mentioned, was the immediate origin of the triggers. I used to have the capacity to think on and speak about distressing things happening in my life.

After hitting my head, it seemed I couldn't do either. Even the anticipation of what might occur upon considering such things usually was enough to instigate.

JOSHUA HOLMES

• • •

As a general rule, I usually tried to encourage my web design clients to choose a web hosting company (which required a monthly fee), to select Wordpress (my specialty), a template, and then give me the login name and password so that I could customize a site for them. To this day, I don't think I swayed from this set of instructions when working with Adaline.

One afternoon, after The Festive Shore closed for the day, I showed to the country-folk style deli and situated myself at one of the hard, wooden tables within, so that I could guide them through the needed steps to create a site.

"I can manage a monthly charge," she said. "But I would like to keep our current domain name."

"A transfer takes time," I said. "Like a couple weeks, depending on your current host company. But it shouldn't be a problem."

The phone rang, and Adaline rose to take it. She was loud; made a scene; eventually sat down again.

Like so many previous times, I presented a few possible templates. If you could land a pre-existing look that worked, you were a step ahead of the game. For whatever reason, she didn't like that we were starting with a used design, as if it wouldn't be unique in the end.

"I was thinking something like this," I said, showing my computer, which contained a screenshot of a food sales template or theme. "It is geared towards delis and catering."

TRIGGER

Had Adaline owned a mattress store, I would have offered an array of sales and bed-oriented themes, as each company required product/service-specific styling.

"A paid host site will allow me to make this template—any template—exclusive to The Festive Shore, which I believe is what you want.

"A new corporate identity would go there." I pointed at the top of the screen. "Perhaps along the side. It would really modernize things. The current outdated logo would be replaced with something fresher.

"If you'd explain the demographic we're trying to reach that would help," I said. "I imagine young to middle-aged women looking to get married."

"Yeah Chris," Adaline managed. "Don't worry about the men."

"So pastel colors then," I said.

"I was thinking black and gold."

So she wanted minimalist and modern, the antithesis of the current dining area; No block letter signage, no tacky, landscape paintings, no curvaceous cabinetry.

"Any additional thoughts or questions that I can speak to or answer for you?"

The phone rang again. She took it once more. I sensed she was used to dictating the direction of her meetings. *Ridiculous*, I thought.

"I think that'll be all. I'll be in touch."

"I need you to decide on a preferred template if I am to work further on this."

"After my meeting tomorrow."

Right, I thought. *Another meeting.*

I hadn't gathered what I needed, but she had given all she intended to for the time being.

• • •

6
OVERDRESSED

HANK AND I donned our gis beforehand. At the time, we didn't know any better. There was no handbook, and anybody could have made the same mistake.

The study of Kali didn't require a uniform at all. Tae Kwon Do did, but didn't demand you dress at the dojo. Shotokan, as it turned out, asked you dress on-site.

Because we were club members, studying a given skillset, we soon gathered, we weren't to advertise our discipline, no matter how indirectly.

And as we improved, Sensei would also emphasize the importance of keeping our progress under wraps.

But that particular night, there were no secrets. Our naivety was on full display.

"What are you guys doing?" demanded Sensei.

Our subsequent expressions of concern were reflected in all the floor-to-ceiling mirrors, which seemed to elevate the moment's gravity.

"What do you mean, Sir?" I said. "We're ready to start."

ELECTRIC

We stood there at the front door, beltless, eager to begin, but forced to defend an error in front of our peers. It seemed the life-size, pouncing tiger glared down at us from the far wall.

"We have dressing rooms here," said Sensei. "From now on, you change there."

"It's my fault," I said. "We were running late, and my previous teacher didn't mind. I suggested it. Shouldn't have assumed."

"No. You shouldn't have."

"It won't happen again, Sir," I said. "We'll attempt to get here earlier."

A bit embarrassed, Hank and I bowed our heads submissively, went into the small locker room, calmed and collected ourselves, re-tied our uniforms, and then walked back out to locate our respective places.

AFTERWARDS, WE formally met Rahal, the tallest, longtime blackbelt member of the Shotokan Club who exuded a quiet confidence that fit his stature.

"Yeah…wearing your suit in will rustle feathers every time."

"Well. Apparently." I laughed uncomfortably. "I just hope everyone knows it was accidental."

Rahal looked down at me as he rolled up his belt and started dressing.

"Not the way I imagined starting," I continued. "But it was never an issue in my previous study."

"You have studied previously."

"Seven years. Kali, Jiu Jitsu, and Tae Kwon Do."

JOSHUA HOLMES

I dismantled my suit and protective gear, and hopped into my Levis and t-shirt.

"Ah, some cage fighting."

"And stick fighting."

"Different standards."

"For sure."

"Well. Welcome to Shotokan!"

"Thanks." I turned to Hank and smiled. "We can only go up from here, right?"

"Right."

• • •

7
DISTRACTION

AT TEMPSTAR again, I briskly walked over to Greta's brimming desk with my head held high. I'd done my best since she brought up my distraction to act anything except, but—as I'd mentioned before—I knew I was transparent. Even with a veneer, I wore my true feelings on my sleeve.

I actually took pride in this quality, as it had served me well in more cases than not. Most people—friends and clients—embraced my authenticity, regardless of the approach. But ask me to hide what ailed me for a time, and it eventually emerged in a manner I later regretted.

Beside the fact that Greta was smart, and, without question, already sensed my facade, I also wanted to be true to myself.

TRIGGER

And yet I didn't want to burden Greta.

"I'M THE one who suggested trying a different restaurant of your choosing," I said after she opted for the rather dim Primanti Bros. "But I'm glad you didn't go for The Festive Shore."

"Are you kidding, Chris?" said Greta. "Considering how they've treated you? I couldn't!"

"Well, you could have," I said. "But you didn't. So thank you for being so sweet to me."

My quaint, composed, strong girlfriend momentarily lost her cool, growing defensive for me.

"The silent treatment from that woman!" said Greta, an expression of disbelief on her face. "What gall!"

I shrugged my shoulders, unable to offer more. "I know, right?"

The numerous celebrities and athletes painted in the mural above looked down at us, seemingly amused yet equally clueless.

"Whatever happened to cooperating with class?"

"In any case," I said. "I personally decided, on principle, not to dine there as much, because it might have a bearing on things."

"Any more, perception is everything, isn't it, hon?"

"In many cases, yes," I said. "And who knows what opinions she's formed about me."

"I assume that's part of what's been bothering you," said Greta.

"I have been over-analyzing the whole situation, lately, I admit."

"But there's something else troubling you. I can feel it!"

Wow. She was persistent!

• • •

8
EVOKED

WHEN I felt lonely, violated, or upset in grad school, and nobody in the debate club—Michael, Linda, John, or Alex—could help, I'd go into downtown State College, to the bookstore, peruse some antiquated novels, and get some counsel from Sam, the wise bookstore owner and my friend who proudly sported a war injury and dreads.

Years later, Stone, relaxed Starbucks manager and friend, had kind of acted that part in York, when we started bowling together. And after that, Hank and Foster stepped in to a degree.

I considered how fortunate I'd been to have these people—how much emptier I could have felt without them—but also how, upon calling Wellspan Neurology, Mary Grace's plausible answer evoked a momentary sadness that these friends usually covered.

At first, it was a distress about her reactions, but then it was a general disappointment over the entire mess that had emerged between us.

It still gnawed at me in the recesses of my brain that my crush on the blue-eyed blonde had lasted for so long, that I'd wasted time and energy on someone other than Greta, and seized mightily in the process.

And yet I hadn't done anything wrong, so the melancholy she invited had less to do with any kind of regret, and mostly reflected how—even after healing—the past could sting.

ELECTRIC

AND SO I did my best to expect a sting. I imagined it would make the calls easier. The clinic visits were few and far between, and I escaped contact last time, but the calls concerning medicine acquisition had increased tenfold, since every year the government played a larger, god-like role in my healthcare.

"I realize the pharmacy usually does this," I said. "Just trying to expedite things."

"A priority fax was just sent to your insurance company."

"And there's nothing else I can do," I said. "I am nearly out of my meds. It's important I get it ASAP."

"That should force a 24-hour turnaround."

"So I should expect a call tomorrow," I said.

"That's cutting it close."

"I'll be sure to tell the POCA," said the secretary.

"Will have her call you as soon as we hear back."

I really did want to trust these people. But I'd witnessed first hand what happens to some in the medical community after a prolonged exposure to illnesses beyond their control. They built walls of their own. An immunity emerged.

How did I know the right POCA would find out the information I sought? Would Rhys try, or would Mary Grace interfere? And in a way that was beneficial?

• • •

JOSHUA HOLMES

9
ANTICIPATION

So I briefly mentioned the ever-increasing role of anticipation in the moments preceding a trigger. I have a few things I'd like to add.

I don't know about you, but I tried to use the word "eager" when I was excited about something, and "anxious" when I was uptight. And I'd use one or the other term here if I could categorize "anticipation" positively or negatively.

However, I could be feeling good or bad at any given time, and subconsciously overwhelmed, and—out of nowhere—get sucker punched by a trigger.

There were periods when I could ward off the trigger for a little. The sensations in my eyes, by then, though, were so regular and strong, I couldn't help but return to the feeling of the impending attack. I had considered the impact of excess worry or concern, of whether controlling them, or leaving behind the emotions altogether would resolve everything.

I especially wished for this on the days when my schedule was adjusted against my will, when I had five and six back-to-back seizures, and—out of wisdom and mercy for those around me—I chose to stay at home so everybody might escape a public scene.

• • •

Everyday—even on the days I had to stay home because of a trigger—I continued to pick away at Adaline's website, to move the content over to a different host, and enhance the overall

TRIGGER

look. To this day, I believe I created something that blows away The Festive Shore's old site.

I moved the pages and the menus, customized the fonts, and replaced the low-resolution photos with temporary, high-resolution ones.

For a while, I stopped by the deli to make conversation with and skim some ideas off of her staff, to see if I missed or could learn anything new. But when that yielded nothing, I finished doing that.

Despite Adaline's neglectful business practices, I reached out to her to try and build rapport, and to better understand the growing disconnect.

"Adaline," I said into the phone. "Chris here. Do you have a minute?"

"Actually," she said. "I'm very busy."

"I'm calling to touch base. It's been a while."

"Yes. I know," she said. "I was just going to email you some photos. My daughter took them."

So I could add more photos.

She'd brought up her daughter before, how she put out terrific design work. I was always open to new approaches if, in fact, they were fresh.

I hoped this didn't turn into some kind of competition. For, in the end, family ideas usually trumped those of the freelancer. As the saying went, blood was always thicker than water.

So far, everything about this project felt wrong.

• • •

JOSHUA HOLMES

10
MAINTENANCE

HANK AND I started studying all the core components of Shotokan, properly dressed and enthused, soon thereafter. And, once in a groove, twice a week at that!

To reap the benefits, I quickly learned, it required a different level of commitment and energy than I had ever previously known. Mastering the details was vital.

I appreciated this, because I loved succeeding at seemingly insurmountable challenges, defying norms and expectations. And Hank told me he did too, but, I gathered, for unique reasons of his own.

I'll speak for myself here, but, initially, the study seemed so demanding that I doubted myself, wondering some nights if, just maybe, I'd bitten off more than I could chew.

I asked this most frequently when, originally, because we were brand new, Hank and I had to mop the floors together following an intense night of kumite' (sparring).

"You know, Hank," I said under my breath. "When I signed up for this, I didn't know I was getting into maintenance for a living."

To top it off, if you were going to mop, you had to follow a certain technique that entailed pushing the massive cloth swab parallel to your co-worker's own, heaving forward with control and in unison.

"Right," said Hank, who had to be equally exhausted.

"I suppose it teaches further discipline to the kids," I said. "And forces the adults to lead."

ELECTRIC

"Right."

"But immediately after class?" I said. "My body is burning right now!"

For the first few months—until new members joined and replaced us as Shotokan virgins—we mopped the floors as thoroughly as we could, shook the dirt from the cloth outside, then returned them to the closet.

I often wondered whether Sensei used the maintenance responsibility as a means to measure student commitment and analyze work ethic.

If nothing else, the dojo—after many years in existence—still looked brand new. Perhaps cleaner than any other I'd visited.

"SEVERAL YEARS back," said Rahal, recalling history as he put the cleaner back under the sink. "They built this place with their own hands."

"So everyone has said," I noted. "It is a nice place, nicer than the barn, I hear."

We looked across the field at the former training site each night we practiced. It was a decent construct, I thought, but, then again, I'd never been inside, and it was inevitably aged in comparison to the current school.

"Air conditioned, for one."

"That is a plus."

"Much nicer, for sure."

"Well, Hank and I swept. I will sleep good tonight."

"You did surprise us. Coming again."

"What do you mean?"

"We didn't expect you'd be back," added Rahal, contented the trash was still empty, returning to the locker. "You started on a demanding night, after all."

"It was tough, yes, but nothing that would cause me to quit."

"Me neither," said Hank.

• • •

11
SET JAW

So I was guilty of stalling, I admit. I pushed off divulging my distractions to Greta, with the exception of repeating the regulars: Work, Epilepsy, and karate. Days passed, but I could tell my girlfriend wanted me to share more.

I was interested to see whether she would note my hesitance and respect my desire for space, or if she'd pursue a response out of a need for control or frustration.

I already knew she was strong and resilient, a fiercely loyal friend, that she'd already handled herself with grace, but some things you could only learn with time and through experience.

For days, I watched her bite her tongue about all manner of topic, her slight underbite exaggerated. But her set jaw was most apparent when I didn't reciprocate about my hidden concern the way she wanted.

OVER LUNCH on a different day. At Jersey Mike's, I believe. I learned more about Greta and passivity, in general.

TRIGGER

I took a seat, and said to Greta, "I haven't figured this place out yet. Food's good. Prices are outrageous. And it's packed!"

"It is that," said Greta. "I think we managed the last seat."

CNN quietly flashed deceiving headlines on the overhead television, and a stereo with blown speakers roared, muffling most conversation, encouraging customers to pay, eat, and leave.

"Like who is the target audience?"

A stream of African Americans, Hispanics, and Caucasians—meandering in no particular order from the entrance all the way to the front cash register—waited their turns in line.

"Good question."

"Don't get me wrong," I said. "I like it."

"I know you do."

"And I think you do, right?"

"Yes Chris. It is nice every now and again."

"McDonalds seems to have captured the minority. Starbucks has the rich majority group. But this brings in every class and subgroup. It really does break all the classic marketing trends."

"They are called trends for a reason," said Greta.

"I suppose so," I conceded, considering all that had changed in the past several years. "But it still doesn't make sense to me."

I watched Greta's eyes narrow, her jaw harden, and I knew I said something that hit a nerve.

"Give me a few minutes. I could tell you what else doesn't make sense to me."

She hadn't overtly said anything about my stall tactics, so in the next few moments, I let her unload about how they bothered her.

Truth of the matter was, I could rid of that hardened jaw by fully trusting Greta, with a little courage and self-disclosure.

The real question, though: How soon would I get there?

• • •

12
UNKNOWN

MARY GRACE did not pick up after the other POCAs like she once did, because, apparently, Wellspan Neurology re-assigned her to another Physician's Assistant (PA) with different expectations. But that didn't mean she didn't interfere.

From experience, I knew she'd only endure ineptitude so long before she took steps of her own.

How sensitively she now resolved a matter was beyond me, though, as she wasn't the caring angel I previously knew her to be. That said, the status of my meds was still unknown.

So I awaited that supposed 24-hour turnaround, hopeful I'd get immediate insurance company approval, but dreading who might have involved herself.

The hours moved more slowly than I thought possible, and my stomach contents burned like hot coals at the back of my throat.

I'M NOT sure why I assumed the insurance company would have my back. They'd proven through past encounters—regarding thousands of dollars in ambulance charges—that they didn't mind making life hard.

ELECTRIC

And they'd prove the fact again when they denied assistance to Rhys, followed by Mary Grace, and forced me to interact with my ex.

"So let me get this straight, Mary Grace," I said, totally disgusted. "For the past, what? Fifteen years? Someone in that office has called on my behalf. And now you aren't allowed to call for your patient?"

"You're not my patient," said Mary Grace. "I'm helping Rhys."

"Whatever Mary Grace. Point is, it doesn't make sense."

"This is on your insurance company. Not us."

"Nobody is blaming anyone."

"I'm just relaying information."

"So where do we go from here then? Can Rhys guide me now, or are you at the helm?"

"You have to call and appeal."

"I'm out of my meds today."

And so, what began as a relatively small, inner-conflict grew into a persistent problem without a foreseeable solution.

• • •

13
THE UNSETTLING

ANOTHER CHOICE most people enjoy, but, in my case, often initiated a trigger, was that which led to the repeat discussion of a setback or discouragement or anything particularly edgy.

More often than not, it wasn't the actual existence of said emotions that set things into motion, or even its rehashing, but rather, during conversation, what my partner (anybody talking to me, really) suggested I ought to feel, or the recommended alternate manner in which I should address an issue.

Not that I was opposed at all to different methods. I opened myself to this as a student for 15 years. And as a contracted employee, after that. Prided myself for it, actually. To this day, I love widening my knowledge base.

Unfortunately, the notion of deliberating and deciding again between multiple perspectives and/or approaches after arriving at the fact that a given topic was especially significant and disturbing or exciting was too much. I suppose the mere mention of facing immediate difference unsettled me.

• • •

THE DAILY unsettling in my gut due to Adaline's sporadic communication practices lingered. Every day, I prayed for peace about it. But random exchanges, no payment, and a blatant dismissal of my hard work ate at me.

I probably advised myself more than anyone to just let it go, since I didn't know what exactly was proper protocol when you were taken advantage of. *You can buckle under the abuse*, I thought. *Or you can stay focused.*

And, at some point, I finally decided to continue with my daily routine. When in doubt, I resorted to the productive path that kept me occupied.

The photos weren't bad. I had to give Adaline's daughter that much. And they did spruce the site up once I mixed and matched a few.

TRIGGER

But I was a collaborative designer. In other words, I typically worked alongside my clients to achieve a desired outcome. In my opinion, teamwork yielded the best result. After a long day of experimentation, I'd wonder, What photos feel most vibrant to Adaline?

In this instance, I'd never really know if making improvements mattered. Aside from the random, confusing emails, I had no clear idea of her expectations.

Frankly, I was starting to wonder if she had any at all.

• • •

14
TIME & REPETITION

EVEN AS Hank and I grew in the area of maintenance, we inevitably grew as martial artists, too. I could confidently announce we were becoming tidy, self defenders.

Each day of study demanded physical and mental strength one could only accrue with time and repetition. Over and over again, we invested energy into the same moves, getting more comfortable with it all.

Our bodies—mine specifically—didn't catch on the way we always wanted, but the span and practice did improve our propensity for observation and adaptation. It was enough to keep us pushing.

In this field, perfection didn't exist, and results were hard to see. If you didn't look at the effort through a long-term lens, it was easy to get disheartened. A man who operated on high standards, I constantly had to reset.

JOSHUA HOLMES

Once I was personally reset, I could embrace the instructors' constantly imparted tweaks. I didn't know if Hank had to reset, as he seemed to take it better than me, but his resilience impressed me.

We had to display our resilience when we partnered up to repeatedly block, punch, and kick on the small and large, bright blue bags.

"GOOD POSTURE men!" Sensei paced before us. "Shoulders back! So important!"

I grimaced, silently scolding myself, and stood straighter.

Hank and I stood opposite each other. I moved into Front Stance (Zenkutsu Dachi), preparing to practice my favorite kick, a Roundhouse (Mawashi Geri).

"Chris. Widen your stance!"

"Yes sir."

Wouldn't I have done it already if I knew better?

I raised my arms, and landed an arcing kick straight into the bag, Hank fell back and was thrown off-balance.

"Protect your body!" I adjusted.

"Both feet facing forward." I shifted.

"Toes tucked." I bent.

"Knee up and out!" I lifted and thrust.

"All the way through." And I extended.

I did my best to keep up, to fit in, to improve like those around me, to avoid a scene. But I was different. And the criticism was prevalent.

"Hank," said Sensei. "Withstand the blow."

"Yes Sir."

ELECTRIC

I wiped sweat from my brow. Hank followed suit. Tonight had been demanding. Intense. Another night for the resilient.

"JUST DON'T quit," said Rahal, the congenial black belt, in the locker room, which smelled strongly of bleach. "Keep it up. We still haven't got it exactly right. And we've been at it a while longer."

"For sure," I said, straddling the lone bench. "I'm just hard on myself."

"You worked your butt off out there!" said Rahal, opening his locker with a grin. "You too, Hank!"

"Thanks," said Hank from the corner. He once again would make it outside before me.

"I can tell you're both getting better."

Hank smiled, acknowledging the compliment.

I undressed and stuffed my gi and cup in the gym bag. And then grabbed my shirt and pants. "I appreciate the encouragement. That was a critique and a half tonight."

Rahal batted a free hand at the door, "Ahh. The critiques won't stop. Might seem harder, in fact."

"Right," said Hank, carrying his small bag, heading out.

"Good to know," I said, securing my regular attire, jewelry and cap. "Let's hope I get used to it."

"It's to make you better is all."

Inside, I knew he was right.

• • •

15
TOO SMART

HOW SOON would I get to that place of no fear, of full trust in and disclosure to Greta? As it turned out, not immediately, but more quickly than I originally thought.

As tired and bothered as Greta was—evidenced by her regular, sharp expression, and not-so-subtle probes, mind you—I was equally tired of initiating "the look". It was cute in a way, yes, but knowing what emotions lay behind the expression also upset me, and forced me to re-consider the disability issues that were at the heart, and how damaging was protecting privacy.

"You're too smart to think I wouldn't notice or inquire about what troubles you, Chris."

We'd arrived at that point—an impasse—where the normal lunch formalities weren't even cutting it. Nor were the random restaurant changes. And I could forget all demographic analysis. She would jump right into the divisive matter we both struggled to ignore.

"You're right," I tried. "I've spent a long time processing. Keeping things to myself."

"Former counselor, too," she said. "A communication specialist. Not to throw the obvious in your face, but you know how this is supposed to go down."

"I have an idea."

"Well then?"

"Isn't that how it always goes?" I said. "The person academically schooled gets schooled by life later on?"

"Seriously hon," said Greta. "What could possibly be so bad that you can't share it with me?"

Only that every time I've grown close to someone, they've been scared away by my condition.

"You're right, Greta."

"This is the last time I'll ask," she said, shaking her head. "Too smart, love. You're too smart."

I *was* too smart. I heard the ultimatum loud and clear.

• • •

16
APPEAL

"BEFORE YOU say anything," I said to the insurance rep. "I've already been given the runaround. Have heard all the one-liners."

Her voice sounded reserved, her tone caring and confident, causing me to imagine a serious, patient woman who knew her limits, but who wasn't afraid to try.

"Well I'm sorry to hear that."

"You and me both."

"I do see you've called about this before."

"Yep," I said. "And I've been told everything under the sun. That the doctor has to provide justification. Advised only to talk to the pharmacist. And that I need to file an appeal. Which, I understand, will take a month. Got that."

"Just let me pull up your records, Chris," she said. "It will only take a minute."

"That's fine, ma'am," I said. "But, bottom line, I'm just about out of meds. I've been going in circles, and I need someone who will fight for me, who will attempt to figure this out on my behalf."

"I will do my best, Sir."

"That's all I ask."

I gave her all the phone numbers at my disposal, to the various doctors and pharmacists. And she took them, claiming she would make a few calls for me.

"I'll be in touch after I've reached out to these folks. Will try to get that medicine to you by day's end."

BLESSING THAT the experienced insurance rep was, Mary Grace squashed her efforts, and turned the whole situation inside out, pinning the blame everywhere except on Wellspan Neurology.

"I did talk to the rep," said Mary Grace. "And she explained everything."

"Nothing new that I hadn't already gone over with you guys." Rhys hadn't talked to me since the day of the appointment, and had been pushed aside, I assumed, since she didn't know my history as well, and didn't make headway with my insurance company.

"The rep talked to your PA, too."

"And what did she say they want?"

"The fact you're out of meds isn't the issue," she said. "Neither is the type. It's the amount. And they are still requesting legitimate proof you require it."

"My records have already been sent!"

She sighed, obviously annoyed. "I know that."

ELECTRIC

"Twenty some odd years worth, at that!"
"Uhuh."
"I just don't get it," I said. "What do I have to do? Go into Status?"
"I don't know. But we've already complied to the extent we can."
"So you're out of answers."
"Totally out."
 Was it that, or did she even care in the first place?

• • •

17
ROLES

SINCE I expounded on the roles of thought, talk, anticipation and repetition on triggers, I felt the need to mention one other thing. During this time, cognitively addressing problems ushered in electrical storms. And yet a purposeful quiet about an upsetting matter did the same exact damage; To internalize it somewhere up front precipitated an eventual show when it manifested in one private or public form or another.

That said, a half year ago now, I arrived at a place where I threw caution to the wind, and I started digging through my own personal make up. I was born with choice, and it bothered me that I couldn't choose what topics to address and avoid without provoking a physical assault.

Minus medicine or further experimentation, was it possible to eliminate the underlying causes of triggers? If I knew the derivation was emotional, would all this stop with an emotional fix?

JOSHUA HOLMES

So much of karate was mastery of the mind and the body, reaching a degree of peace and self control, exerting energy only when necessary, no longer expending it negatively, in excess. More importantly, my Christian belief system echoed similar instruction, encouraging universal refinement in order to live in and like Jesus.

Would emotional control limit the seizure origin to a certain sector of my brain? Could I overcome the stimulus that was typically considered out of reach?

Deep down, I was convinced my thought had merit.

• • •

"I CAN'T CHRIS," said Adaline dismissively, confirming how little merit she placed on me.

"It's just been crazy busy this whole month. Can't meet this week."

"Uhuh," I said, falling back on one of Hank's lines. "Right."

"Perhaps at another time."

"Okay," I said, raising my eyebrows. *How do you sleep at night?*

By now, I'd done everything by the book. I'd created the majority of the site, I'd sent over an invoice, and if I lived a life consumed by fairness and money, I could have pursued their absence. But I didn't.

I'd never been treated so poorly, so I was past Adaline's thoughts of me. I hadn't been to the deli in ages, and I didn't plan to return.

A new Starbucks with comfortable chairs and an airy ambiance had gone up across the street, so they would get all my business now. The biggest questions I kept asking myself, however, were: Should I go ahead and shut down the page? Make the past the past?

TRIGGER

The site was connected to my email, and only still existed because I didn't take steps to expire it. I spent hours developing it. And I refused to act out of spite, even if The Festive Shore and its employees hadn't expressed interest in what I'd done for them.

You never knew what might happen in the months to come, and I wasn't about to eliminate a hypothetical opportunity. I supposed she could approach me at some future juncture. And then I'd have to decide whether or not to oblige.

On the other hand, perhaps the Lord had shut down the whole thing to spare me. I recalled other times when He'd done the same.

I admit, I reflected often on the injustice, and there are still days when I look back stunned on what transpired, and I wonder why.

• • •

PART TWO

18
NARROW ESCAPE

MY BODY hung dangerously for all to see over the side of the brown arm chair, and my face tilted unnaturally, slightly reflecting off the coffee-colored, hexagonal table tucked tightly against the windowsill. The tan, tile baseboards seemed to reach up for me like a child wanting a parent in my vulnerability, only to shoo me away as I shook violently for the second time at the new Starbucks that day.

"I just found him like that," said a scared, brunette, college girl worriedly tapping a cell phone screen. "Twisted up and breathing hard."

"Thank you, dear," said Vera, the current, chunky store manager. "I'll take it from here."

JOSHUA HOLMES

That couldn't be good.

"I called for an ambulance."

A jolt of fear jerked me. *Please no!*

I couldn't pin the seizure on a phone call from an Asian telemarketer this time, a fake FBI agent, but I could again blame a trigger, and one that gave me no warning.

This trigger was unique in that it attacked a couple times without my having even known it.

Memory loss a past issue, it somewhat bothered me. And only after re-living the moments could I deduce the origin.

It was pretty busy that day, but there were two of us competing on the phone for personal conversation space, mine business-related, the brunette, college girl beside me assessing a dating matter.

I looked at the girl hard, conveying displeasure, to no avail. The silence and separation I needed in the moment seemed increasingly implausible.

I achieved a severe degree of claustrophobia, yet continued to posture for the better talk, shifting in my seat, trying a stronger cadence in my voice. Let it go, I eventually told myself. It's not worth it.

That was the last I remembered.

FAST FORWARD like an hour. The next snippet
I woke to was chaotic, to say the least. I didn't see myself shaking, although I felt I was stuck and synonymously in motion.

I heard a lot of "It's okay", "Everything will be fine", and "There, there, now." Someone petted me like a dog, as I twitched and leaned forward to gasp.

TRIGGER

"Oh dear," said Vera. "He's shaking again."

What? I thought. *Again?*

Moments after I told myself the phone competition wasn't worth it, I vaguely recalled begging a nearby person to call off the ambulance. And I thought I remembered someone promising me they would.

And yet, in the very space I regularly worked, a tall bed on wheels lurked, the glint of the aluminum supports blinding me.

For the next several minutes, I tried to catch my breath. The room spun, but then suddenly it slowed.

I tried to speak.

"I already said I didn't want an ambulance!"

"The first time, you said you didn't, Chris," said Vera. "The first time."

"What are you saying?"

"This is your second seizure in the last two hours."

"Oh," I said. "I didn't know."

"So the paramedics are here."

I shook my head, exhausted. *Why?*

"No..."

"Yes."

IT WAS a narrow escape. That's the way I saw it. But this time I had a little help from my teacher. Next door, Greta was working and couldn't get away. I mean, she got there as fast as she could, but not nearly as fast as Sensei. That's right, I said Sensei.

Between the first and second seizure, he later explained, we talked, and I expressed my angst about Greta's late arrival, the seizures, and the ambulance workers. Also nearby, he made the special trip to help me out.

"I don't want them here!" I said. "I want to leave!"

Big hands on my shoulders, Sensei said, "Just breathe. You're angry."

"All this because of a stupid trigger!"

"Just try to calm down, Chris."

"I know," I said. "But it's just wrong. All of this!"

Again he regarded me with those steely, blue eyes.

I stared back evenly, quietly, my frustration brimming and ready to spew any moment.

"In and out. Let it go."

I did my best, and looking back, it helped me endure, to stay controlled.

It took forever to convince the EMTs, to defeat their abuse, but when Greta showed—against their wishes—I eventually got up and left with her.

I breathed deeply with all my might, furiously shaking my head all the way home.

• • •

19
HARDER

SUBTLETY ABOUT the study and craft continued to be a major theme as Hank and I pushed ahead in the martial arts. And not just subtlety; Sensei encouraged a silence; and, some nights, he demanded secrecy, especially of the higher belts.

ELECTRIC

Never so much, however, as he did on the nights preceding testing. Hank and I knew we could test every four months, like the majority did, but the reality of showcasing our knowledge base and abilities before our black belt superiors and peers really sunk in when Sensei reminded us of our responsibilities.

"Line up!" he said. "As most of you guys know, rank testing is approaching."

Some of the kids cheered, others grimaced. I didn't flinch, since I was uncertain, a little nervous, and also excited to work even harder and execute. I couldn't read Hank's mind.

"Know your kicks. Know your stances. Know your blocks. Know your punches. And your forms."

Sensei sequentially assembled and enacted a spur of the moment combination of kicks, stances, blocks, and punches, visually demonstrating what we ought to do.

"We want you to know the Japanese terminology, also."

The whole class spent the next few minutes attempting to respond off the cuff to Japanese prompts, so that it became further ingrained in their memories.

"If you confidently show us what you've studied for months, you should all do fine."

Hank and I had come this far. We didn't want to stop progressing now.

Because testing day drew near, Rahal was careful about what he said in and beyond the locker room. To me, it came off kind of rude, aloof perhaps, was humbling, and yet it added a mysterious dimension to the exam in question.

I wondered whether or not Sensei told Rahal about our unfortunate encounter outside the dojo; whether a retelling of my seizure added to his cautious air.

There were plenty of platitudes, like there usually was in the locker room. But they were especially surface during this time. Just as I was getting accustomed to locker room talk too!

"So you guys ready?"

"As ready as a clueless white belt will ever be," I said, grinning. Hank agreed.

"You'll be in and out."

"Since we can't watch the higher belts test," I finished. "I remember."

"Just take all of Sensei's advice, and you will both do well."

"That's the plan."

"Good luck, Chris! Good luck, Hank! See you then!"

• • •

20
TURNING THE CORNER

I WAS MORE accepting of my situation now, but I continued to wonder if it was realistic to ask someone to ignore the "out of control" side of me, or, alternately, to request they assume the whole package.

Like I said though, already, the good news was that Greta had stayed thus far. She had seen me in my serious, intellectual state, in my creative writing state, my design state, and at my worst, in my distraught state, and in my seizure and post seizure stupors. I had, however, exhausted my processing time.

That awkward silence between people had replaced Greta's hard jaw and filler conversation we both relied on at first. And, for me, it had grown so unbearable I secretly wished for the light lunches I used to have with Foster Monroe. In the worst moments of passivity, I even imagined taking an extended trip with him in his truck.

It wasn't long afterwards that I felt prompted. Like a guilt-ridden schoolboy responsible for throwing chalk at the teacher, under the watchful eye of an assuming tattletale, I finally blurted out a confession.

"I'm ready," I said. "I don't want you frustrated with me anymore, and I don't need to carry this a minute longer."

We had made it all the way to the Rt. 30 Olive Garden. Not for the initial reasons I thought a different place might help, but hey, what could you do?

I had a few nervous, aural sensations in my eyes, but nothing trigger-worthy quite yet.

Before another salad, Greta said, "I'm happy to hear that. I don't like feeling exasperated, either."

So I took a deep breath. *I am in the perfect, romantic place to start making reparations*, I thought. *Don't screw it up!*

Because I am the type of conversationalist who prefaces everything first, I offered a couple different angles to my yet-to-be disclosed struggle, which delayed everything some. Greta consumed a little more wine.

"You know how easy it is to work yourself up?" I said. "I mean, not you specifically, universally speaking, how people can do more damage to themselves than those around them can?"

"People can be self-destructive."

"I guess what I'm trying to say," I said, briefly glancing overhead at the black ceiling lamp. "Is that I was turning into that person. Riling myself up. Getting consumed over the past and about the 'could bes'."

"It's easy to do," she said. "I've been there."

"Glad I'm not alone."

"But if I hear you correctly," Greta finished. "You were there, thinking about us."

I nodded honestly, a massive weight lifted off my shoulders.

• • •

21
ROADBLOCK

AT THIS point, I decided, whether or not Mary Grace was out of ideas or cared at all about my situation was of little consequence. To wish for the best, with our past, would prove emotional and naïve. And to stand by idly would waste precious time and leave me without meds, unprotected.

She was one heck of a roadblock, and—as only one of millions driving on the highway of life—I just had to press the pedal to the metal, and go out around her.

ELECTRIC

If my past offered a reliable reference, I knew that, once I took the risk, moving past my impediment, an alternate life choice usually emerged, identifying hurdles as the temporary challenges they were.

One way or another, I knew all would see Mary Grace for the hindrance she was.

It was time to rustle feathers, to create my own options. I had to start moving multiple wheels at once, to weed out the uninformed, and locate the people of character who looked at me as more than a "medical unit", and cared about my welfare.

"Since you're out of ideas, Mary Grace," I said. "Let me talk to someone who has some."

"I'm in charge now because Rhys…"

"What?" I interrupted. "She ran out of ideas?"

"Well, Chris," said Mary Grace. "Yes. But it was a little more than that."

"How much more complicated could it be? She didn't communicate ideas that weren't there!"

"In any case…"

"So put me on the phone with the doc."

"She's busy with other patients now."

"Mary Grace," I said. "I'm tired of this 'I will speak to her for you and call you back' business."

"It's protocol."

"Not when there's an emergency. Not when you don't have answers after several tries. Not when info gets lost in translation."

"Ok Chris. I'll see what I can do."

You could do a lot, I thought. *If you really wanted.*

"I'm on a deadline, Mary Grace. Surely you get that," I said. "Please just ask the doc to call me."

• • •

22
RECOVERY

THE SHOCK of the initial seizure return had waned, and yet the recovery period following my most recent duo of seizures offered up time to ponder what transpired.
Regardless of how quickly I started life again, how 'normal' everything appeared on the surface, trauma was trauma, and—for healing—I required reflection.

So, although my brain and body were exhausted and I should have just rested, I still processed.

Blinds drawn, I sat on the floor against my second couch in the quiet, and believe it or not, I had a few epiphanies.

As I've already disclosed, I had a pretty solid grasp on the mental and emotional facets of triggers.

I couldn't ignore that I seized whenever the subconscious moved.

But I hadn't fully grasped perhaps the most mysterious components of my condition: how certain outside stimuli jarred all of my senses, the world itself ultimately acting as a trigger wherever I went.

The excess sensory stimulation wasn't necessarily new. In fact, it was commonplace for me, and for many others with Epilepsy. An interest in the way it occurred, and in a personal capacity to overcome it did surface, however.

And if I could somehow acquire understanding, and see some order in the subliminal, perhaps I could arrive at an orderly explanation for the sensory overload.

• • •

IT WAS ironic. To consider sensory overload while Adaline was still in the picture. If anything, she offered the opposite—sensory deprivation—which left me reaching for a happy medium, a filler project hard to come by right now.

As was her norm, she didn't even show to the same meeting she arranged for us, following the last cancellation. I imagined because, in her words, she was "too busy". Days passed, and it grew clear she didn't plan to respond to the invoice I sent her, either. And let's just say it didn't improve my overall opinion of her.

How many times had I given her the benefit of the doubt? Numerous times! More than enough opportunity to redeem herself, that's for sure.

I tried to entirely walk away from the project, but it was hard.

Even as she showed and communicated with less frequency, I thought about the product I created more often. Not because it would amount to anything; Instead, because a perfectly functional design had gone to waste. Or so it seemed.

• • •

JOSHUA HOLMES

23
STUDY

HANK AND I randomly asked each other—over the phone, in person, and at stop lights in the car—what certain Japanese words meant, and what moves corresponded with given terms as the big day crept up on us. And yet the actual act of studying fell on us individually, and we both addressed the task separately.

As was the case ten years ago, when I studied Kali and Jiu Jitsu in State College, I (all current, paying club members, too) had exclusive access to York Shotokan Club study material that would help me master vocabulary and more.

Repetition and space were my two strongest allies when studying. I copied and pasted my required data into a word document per one teacher's suggestion, glanced over it every free chance I had, closed my eyes as I repeated everything aloud, and took a walk to give it time to stick. I cycled through the same process as often as possible.

At my request, Hank kindly explained his own process. He spoke to his creation of lists, of a word-to-karate move matching system, and a slightly different yet equally effective memorization technique.

Depending on the night, I felt better or worse about how much I'd soaked up. I found myself blanking on certain words. Especially if I couldn't connect them to clever image associations as reminders.

About those words I managed to correlate with memorable visuals, I didn't worry anymore. I laughed at the inventions, shared them with Hank, and thought, *Perhaps both of us can benefit.*

I did know, from tireless studying in school, however, that—regardless of Sensei's wise advice and of your confidence level—

there came a point when you had to let it go, and trust your brain to kick in under the gun.

I think Hank and I both fell back on this truth.

• • •

24
LIGHTER

WHILE I felt substantially lighter after bearing my soul to Greta, I didn't release the full weight off of my shoulders just yet, and wouldn't until I finished explaining myself, and then endured the entirety of her response, good or bad.

You could watch a million films depicting two people in love returning to one another to mend fences, and still not experience or comprehend the intensity of the moment. Unprepared for my own sensitive response, I pondered this, even as my insides shuddered and I tried to better self disclose.

Another thing films failed to show was how the exchange was rarely contained to one scene. I had originally hoped to keep our new dialogue going during our lunches, but it spilled over into multiple settings—our breakfasts, coffees, and dinners together.

"I have been stressed about all the other things, social, physical, and medical, for real," I said one evening over delivered Chinese food. "But in varying degrees they're always there. It was the concerns about us, as you said, that bothered me most, and had me beyond uptight."

"So that was your 'beyond uptight' mode?" said Greta, mixing chicken, noodles, and soy. "I perceived stress, but not that level."

"I suppose I'm not the dramatic type," I said, pointing at my Mandarin Chicken. "Although I absolutely love this stuff."

"An accurate statement, I'd say."

"The chicken actually looks and tastes real."

"As opposed to some other places around town, you mean. Whose meat is questionable."

One of her best qualities was her open-mindedness. Some women had this "my way or the highway" mentality, which put a real damper on the communication process.

I grabbed for some Chinese noodles. "By now, you know I'm a planner."

"You operate best that way."

"And I know you are an organized, business woman yourself."

"I like to think so."

"And you also know I think short-term and long-term."

"Yes."

She got up and placed her Won Ton Soup in my fridge for later.

"It's smart to do, I think. Natural, even. And yet the seizures change the outlook," I said. "How it might occur. How it all will transpire."

"Until—if and when—you're healed, they always will be an issue."

I nodded. "So much is contingent on its presence, its absence."

"Like what steps you'll take."

I nodded.

"How long it might take. And with whom."

"The last of which is most important."

• • •

TRIGGER

25
CLASH

I HAD SPENT years acquiring medicine whenever I was low on supply, and clashing with the powers-that-be to collect the right kinds and amounts of anti-convulsants. I was experienced in it.

Enough to know Mary Grace would either drop the ball entirely, or the doctor would get a message when it was convenient and take her time getting back to me.

I've waited up to forty minutes in my doctor's office while she mingled and laughed outside the door just feet away; At home, I've waited until office hours were up, only to rely on another provider to come through for me.

Remember, in their eyes I'm not priority. I don't say this with a victim mentality. The fact of the matter is that I'm just one 'medical unit' of many. And yet it didn't and will never deter me.

I've said as much already, but it is important for people with Epilepsy to bear it in mind when self-advocating. You have to be the match to start a fire of activity, because you are worth it. I knew I was.

So I got off the phone with Mary Grace, didn't anticipate much proactivity from her, and started calling every person and group who had helped me in the past.

Who, specifically, would rise to the occasion and resolve my dilemma was unknown, but—by the time I'd finished—several entities were working towards the same goal for me: medicinal coverage.

I pressed ahead as Mary Grace and the doctors dragged their feet.

"IF I can get enough to hold me over for a few days, it will postpone the seizures long enough, and allow you to make special arrangements."

I must have repeated that phrase a million times. My wrist ached from squeezing my cell phone, and my throat was raw from trying to convince people no coverage could lead to personal harm.

"Oh my. Well we can't have you seizing. Surely something can be done."

Nearly every person I called spoke that platitude.

Making special arrangements, however, required concern and action, which was often in short supply. I hoped for the best, but continued reaching out.

I then added a line that seemed to connect with some. "I need enough to control the triggers."

• • •

26
ILLUSTRATION

MY MIND didn't have to roam far to land on a perfect example to illustrate a sensory trigger. My strongest focal triggers—overstimulation of the eyes—occurred at the dojo, and nine times out of ten when practicing with speed.

They were brought on every night we performed running sessions with somersaults to refine reflexes, and transitioned into jumping jacks or push-ups to build stamina.

What most of the attending students considered regular warm ups were swift actions that induced a strong warning or aura for me.

ELECTRIC

And the only caveat that influenced how suddenly I faced the trigger was how fluidly I perceived and absorbed my surroundings, which, it felt, changed regularly.

Out of shape, I continued running beneath the lights, in circles, jumping headlong into the blue mats, returning to my feet as fast as possible, all the while pushing through a queasy pit in my stomach, trying to beat the trigger.

Sensei clapped his hands, jogging among us, urging us to push ourselves beyond what we thought feasible. If he had any idea what else I was pushing through...

I lasted as long as I could. Sooner rather than later, however, I couldn't keep up, felt weak, and as if I were looking down an endless hallway headed into a bright light. Kind of like that famous scene at the end of *Ghost*, the movie, when Demi Moore looks up at a vivid, ethereal likeness of Patrick Swayze.

I didn't understand how profoundly light and speed combined in a nice gym could bother my sense of sight, but it was only one example. I'll get to some other senses before long.

• • •

As FOR Adaline and The Festive Shore, there was little else to illustrate. If it were somehow a waiting game, and I was acting patently impatient, I could accept her choice to postpone things again and again. But it wasn't a game, I hadn't approached the process any differently, and I hadn't technically gone anywhere.

JOSHUA HOLMES

As I told Greta, I'd stopped eating at The Festive Shore altogether for objectivity and out of principle. But I didn't stop passing the place, didn't stop looking through the deli window.

Most nights, it was dark within. Every now and again I'd get a glimpse of an employee, who would wave. Even so, I'm still not sure why I went out of my way to peer inside.

That was why it came as a major surprise, when, one evening, I saw Adaline on her cell, standing inside, alone, before the meat counter. There, I assumed, for another lame duck meeting.

We locked eyes. She seemed preoccupied, indifferent, phone still at her ear. I thought, *Is that who I think it is?*

I took a second to affirm I had seen correctly, and then quickly looked away, and turned to go, as I had groceries from the store to get home and I wasn't sure either of us wanted to communicate about what hadn't occurred.

Walking into a bitter breeze, I seriously wondered whether I could communicate without exhibiting disgust. While uncertain, I was well aware body language could make a difference.

I would find out as, minutes later, Adaline ran out the door and called my name.

• • •

27
LATE VISUALS

I WOULD ALSO pursue a selection of supplementary visual reference, covering kata and stances and such on the computer, so my compartmentalized brain would see particulars, perhaps even remember.

I didn't get to it right away, however. In fact, I had a late start.

"I've found some especially helpful videos," I told Hank on the last night. "I'm telling you, YouTube is full of stuff!"

"Is that right?"

"Had I realized earlier," I said. "I probably would have watched this stuff after each class. To solidify what we learned that night, you know?"

"Right."

"You have access to a computer at home?"

"Not really."

"What's that mean?"

I asked because, when I needed to do anything computer-related, I just stepped away from Greta, or turned off the news, and Googled the topic or task at hand.

"A family computer," he said. "Not many chances, between Mom, Dad, sister, and brother."

"You couldn't claim it for one night? To study? I'd say that takes precedent over email or social networking."

"I could try."

"I know I'm bringing YouTube videos up like last minute," I said. "But what's the saying? Better late than never? Between the lists and the visuals, it might do the trick!"

"Right."

• • •

JOSHUA HOLMES

28
ABOUT NOW

"**I**'D SAY it's always been about now when my friends and dates of the past up and left me."

I drummed my fingers on the Nittany Pizza table counter after church one Sunday, feeling incredibly exposed.

"I'm not them, though, Chris," said Greta. She was taken by the gluten-free pizza in her right hand, but emphasized her point with a wild wave of her free fingers.

"And that's the point," I said. "You aren't. We seem to have a good thing."

"We seem to have a good thing?"

I surveyed the joint to guarantee our conversation was private. A golf game played softly on a small TV in the corner.

"Bad choice of words," I conceded.

I noted some sauce on her cheek, and got up to grab a few napkins. I then returned and gently wiped her face.

"Good enough that I feel really great about it lasting," I tried once more. "So the point again is?"

"When things feel good—in any event—I also consider the alternative."

I didn't like that I did it now; was doing my best to stop in this context, because I knew you couldn't dwell on the past and also move forward.

"The alternative feeling badly, I assume."

"Usually."

"You can't think like that, Chris!" said Greta. "You just can't!"

ELECTRIC

"Like, is it possible this thing goes off the rails?"

"So that's what you've been so distraught about?"

Now I was exposed and treading dangerous waters. I drummed my fingers and grimaced in my seat.

"Yep," I said. "Guilty."

"None of us know what will happen in the future."

"I can't be 'the Provider'," I said. "The Breadwinner."

The comment was factual, and yet speaking the clichés sounded shallow in my own ears.

"I know that."

"Usually isn't an issue until late in the game."

"Shrinks call legitimizing these concerns 'putting up the walls'."

"I call it bracing myself for the possible."

Greta sucked in a deep breath of pizza-scented air, and looked amidst an array of official, Penn State posters on the walls for a clock that wasn't there.

No matter what you called the apprehension, or how much credence I placed on it, I put myself out there. I was at Greta's mercy, and she could take this where she wanted.

• • •

29
ON CUE

"HELP ME understand, doc," I said. "Help me grasp the hold up."

The round, personable PA—on cue—called hours later with rehearsed notes I recognized as near duplicates of Mary Grace's.

JOSHUA HOLMES

I didn't expect the PA to throw her staff under the bus, but—as the saying goes—I did want her to dot all her I's and cross all her T's.

"Mary Grace claims it's my dosage, not the kind. I already was informed of that."

"Which is accurate." I saw her there sitting on a moving chair, breathing deeply, running her hand through stringy, brown hair, possibly at her wit's end since I often tied her hands, never allowing her to experiment on me.

"But I've also been told by the insurance company they are waiting on proper documentation."

I heard her lean back, the chair squealing in the background. "They've been given all your records."

"Is it possible Mary Grace or Rhys sent over the wrong ones?" I tried. "A general overview that doesn't accurately reflect your own thorough documentation?"

"They have everything," said the doctor, shifting again. "Everything about you."

"And there couldn't be some kind of discrepancy in the database? In the files associated with me, leading to confusion?"

"I'll check," she said. "But I doubt it. I believe your prior-authorizations have been submitted and rejected several times."

"Yes doc. I know. It's why I'm even bothering you."

"Right."

"Well, anything you can do to make sure."

"Alright then, Chris," said the doc. "Is there anything else?"

An uncomfortable silence lingered.

TRIGGER

"No offense, doc," I finally said. "But I'm no closer to understanding why I am being re-directed from one misinformed person to another than when I started."

There was quite a lot more, but expecting answers here was akin to assuming a compliment from a grouch.

• • •

30
PIVOTAL

JUST BEYOND the pull-around order line, and a rough patch of macadam, at McDonalds, there resided a large trash disposal, usually fenced off and meant for restaurant workers and waste management employees. I'd passed it a million times.

One afternoon, on my way to the franchise for a snack, I had a seizure that occurred—at least in my opinion—because of an auditory trigger. The source: a loud garbage truck.

I smelled the vehicle from a distance, yet only looked to my left and upward when I heard repeated, high-pitched warning beeps, and a continuous crunching. The driver seemed nice enough, and encouraged me to keep going. The sound in my ears, though, had done the damage.

I tensed up a little, as it persisted. The duration might have had a bearing, but as I've explained about triggers, their possible explanations are endless and obscure.

I prayed the noise wasn't enough to induce a sensory attack, but the monstrosity was so overpowering in every sense of the word that one minute I was making my way across the parking lot, the next I was pivoting, and then pummeling towards the ground.

After a short stint in the hospital for the McDonalds fall, I made it back to my place, hopeful to finish my day unimpeded, but pretty sure it was just a matter of time before one of my other senses was disturbed.

I hadn't even finished thoroughly examining my newly acquired, external hematoma when my sense of touch started acting up.

On heavy seizure days, I try to continue accomplishing things I otherwise would, and one thing I needed to do was take inventory of my meds. I should clarify: I needed to see if I still had leftovers in my cabinet, and could subsequently use them to hold me over.

In any event, upon finding a few, I began flipping the tabs on my medicine container, which brought on a numbness in my index finger.

I tried to ignore it, since it was initially isolated to a single digit. But the longer I continued flipping the tabs, distributing the extras, organizing my eerily light pill box, the more the numbness spread throughout my fingers.

I vaguely recalled the pillbox flying, falling back, coming to, sweating and heaving amidst a few, tile-strewn capsules.

• • •

I pivoted in more ways than one as Adaline continued after me that evening. First, I circled back on my rear ankle, to again face the deli. And then I pivoted mentally, out of uncertainty and into neutrality.

"Chris!" she said. "Hold up please!"

ELECTRIC

I suppose I shouldn't have been surprised by the plea, as she'd never requested I hurry. But the fact she quickly sought after me was a significant difference.

I won't pretend I immediately thought wonderfully of her. I was shot, and technically shouldn't have even gone out after such a seizure-filled day.

I was cold, my arms burned under the pressure of five, full plastic bags, and her poor track record was pretty consistent. I did stop, though, and manage a courteous, "Yes Adaline. How can I help you?"

She didn't immediately respond, but a few more rushed steps in high heels—a pained, tip-toed jog, it seemed—and she halted a comfortable distance from me. I offered my hand for a semi-formal handshake.

"Hi there."

"You have a lot to carry," she said. "Are you gonna manage it all?"

"It's kinda heavy," I said. "But, yeah, I'll be fine."

"Well, I won't keep you," said Adaline. "But I wanted to express my deepest apologies for how this website attempt has unfolded."

I nodded, tried to smile.

Deepest apologies. Was it genuine? I couldn't tell.

"And things should calm down here in a couple weeks," she continued. "Then we can pick up where we left off."

That sounded optimistic. Almost like a good thing, if I heard correctly. Now, to figure exactly where we left off.

• • •

31
DIRECTIVE

TRAFFIC WASN'T bad the night of the test, and Hank and I got off the exit, covered the three miles, and made it to the dojo perhaps earlier than we ever had.

I think we both were feeling that nervous energy I had on our first day, as the ride over was a little quieter than usual. I sensed a different vibe, and talked less anyway.

Pulling up onto that elevated tract of land, I thought, *How much different will this be from past tests?*

I'd previously participated in heavy, stick-to-stick combat, memorized multiple forms, and even broken boards to climb the belt ladder. Enough to anticipate the unexpected?

Once parked, I grabbed my bag and shut the sedan door. "You ready to do this?"

Hank did the same, and scanned the parking lot, which was packed. "Right."

I can't speak for Hank, but I had studied so hard and watched so many YouTube videos in preparation, my brain had stopped soaking up information. It was as if I'd been given an internal directive: "That will be all!"

I mean, ideally, our grunt work would cover everything, in quantity and quality. Ideally, Hank and I would stand out as deserving.

There was a part of me that recalled my own university testing strategy, though, which I was more likely to apply. I would remember the majority, and lose the excess for a winning result.

TRIGGER

"We should be ok," I said, trying to be positive.

"Right."

And so I think we both entered, up for the challenge, apprehensive about facing something new, yet, either way, ready for the suspense to subside.

• • •

32
CONSIDERATION

DEPENDING HOW you looked at it, you could either conclude Greta and I both already benefitted from the new line of communication, or had a ways to go. Rocky though it was, she coaxed me to open up, and, in time, I reciprocated.

We each—at different points—had turned to passivity, but were uncomfortable in it, eventually emerged from it, and voiced our distaste for it.

And yet I wasn't off base when I said—from this moment on—she could take the matter anywhere she wished. Because she pretty much did.

I wasn't too surprised when she left me hanging for a while. She moved onto talking about work, church, and other relatively small things, I surmised, to allow herself time to consider all I'd said, and make me re-consider feelings that were all-too-real, but nevertheless situational.

You'd never hear me complain about acquired opportunities to self-analyze. As long as it was productive analysis and time well spent.

But our discussion wasn't through, as far as I was concerned. Greta knew where I stood, but I ultimately didn't know where she stood.

So I hoped our talk resumed shortly.

• • •

33
SHIVERS

I GOT A brief call from my primary doctor's office, the secretary inquiring about my recent ER visit, whether I needed to set up a follow-up appointment for my head injury.

It was a nice gesture, I admit, and more than Mary Grace, Rhys, and their POCA crew had done. The PA hadn't gotten back to me about any database issues or employee mistakes. Made me wonder whether she would ever look.

I told the secretary I'd survive, and she didn't object.

Humorously enough, though, I was again referred to Wellspan Neurology if I required further help. Round and round we went.

I shook my head and hung up the phone. Our healthcare system was beyond flawed. Incredible!

The few outdated pills I came across and re-discovered on the floor after the seizure weren't a fix all. They would cover me for a day, at most. And I could expect regular auras, too.

But, until now, trying to persuade the PA and her helpers had yielded zip. Further attempts would probably bring on a faster than low levels.

ELECTRIC

The thought of going through this every month, for years… It gave me shivers.

• • •

PART THREE

34
BURN

"**D**ID YOU fall?" said the wandering man, looking like a parking lot mirage. "Just now, did you fall?"

Of course I'd fallen. I was sprawled out on my back, in behind a dead bush, covered in mulch, to prove it, body tight yet limp and head barely raised to request help.

"A seizure," I managed. "Had a seizure."

Right before my eyes, he looked past me, grimaced, changed course, and walked away. I guessed he could help with a simple fall, but a seizure was too taxing.

JOSHUA HOLMES

I lay my head back down in the mulch under the blinding sun, closed my eyes, and sucked at the air with all my might. Perspiration streamed down my forehead and cheeks.

I was on my way to work at Weis, crossing the road, passing through the lot, when my entire body succumbed to an unknown trigger. A trigger, I should say, that I couldn't classify as subconscious, emotional, or sensory.

It was a physical trigger, I later realized. I hadn't eaten in time, which led to an imbalance inside me. Only after the 2016 concussion had I even noticed the internal disparity that evolved, especially when I waited to quell my hunger.

The memory of the actual fall escaped me, fortunately. And yet I recalled the nearby clothes drop off bin, the plaza direction sign, the vertical Mitzuru Ya flag, and repeated efforts to thrust myself at the median just feet from them all. I recalled burning.

A throbbing lump on the rear of my head, unbelievable muscle spasms in my shoulders, and an indescribable exhaustion was reminder enough of what transpired.

As a strong odor of burnt rubber rose from the pavement and filled my nostrils, I cried out. Help! But I was alone. No one responded. Not even the EMTs. Would this have happened if I consumed lunch an hour earlier?

The heat was sweltering, negating the light breeze overhead, and I could barely think straight as I raised my arms and legs, and observed the damage the hot asphalt had done to them all.

In Postictal, I was short on clarity, but absolutely certain I couldn't bare the scorching elements a minute more.

ELECTRIC

I scanned the full parking lot, everyone there oblivious to the whole ordeal. *I probably could have used a hand today*, I thought.

I located my glasses, cap, and computer bag about five feet away. After brushing mulch from my wounds, I stumbled that way, collected them, and started for home.

• • •

ADALINE'S LATE albeit authentic apology for her poor project handling was a strong reminder to me that if I was to call myself a Christian, I had better willingly offer her forgiveness, as He freely did the same for me.

I again took time to process, yet only because I intended to get over that burn, to the place where I could dismiss the past, and objectively jump back into the website design project that had gone untouched for months.

I did ponder whether or not I should posture, to emphasize the importance of my time and energy, and note that I wouldn't accept poor treatment anymore. But Adaline claimed the overall timing was better now, and seemed to be more interested and engaged.

Before starting again, I did make sure I got paid the first half of what was owed me, and, content with the progress, I then returned to the matter at hand.

"So where would you like me to start," I said. "It's been a while."

"What about the site you were previously assembling?"

"I mean, we've already got a nice looking site up and ready for use," I said. "Although it's hidden from any outside viewer at the moment."

"But you can permit it to be seen."

"I can," I said. If you want me to go ahead and unlock it, and assign your email, I can do that."

• • •

35
CELEBRATION

SHOTOKAN WAS unique in that it was only a four belt system. White. Green. Brown. Black. As opposed to, say, Tae Kwon Do, which had a few more belts and colors.

So while you could acquire additional stripes in your respective color, distinguishing your abilities, in Shotokan you didn't change colors for nearly two years, adding weight to the eventual achievement.

Hank and I were far from "distinctive" at the school, and yet—after all the hype—I think we were proud and relieved to make it through the test. Probably more satisfied our attire wouldn't ever be as barren, that we could finally don a belt.

For me, the belt also reminded me I'd been strong enough to endure relational, physical, spiritual, professional, and general life trials, and still managed to keep a commitment and grow in a separate, healthy discipline.

"Don't know about you, Hank," I said. "But I'm thrilled to have passed that."

"Right."

"I mean, think about it dude," I said. "If we didn't accomplish that, it would've been four more months of beltless training."

"Right."

TRIGGER

"With my history of martial arts training, it would've been super embarrassing for me anyway. Maybe not so much for you, since it's your first time around."

"Right."

In the car, riding home, I secretly celebrated, reflected back on the belting ceremony, after the exam, to the moment Sensei solemnly knotted my belt at my waist, and his black belt cohorts followed after him, individually shaking my hand, repeatedly congratulating me.

"Well, anyway," I said. "That was hard, but it was well worth it."

"Right."

"Congrats bub."

"Thanks," said Hank. "Congrats to you."

I stuck my arms in the air, feigning victory, and laughed. "Woohoo!"

Hank smirked as he drove.

I returned my hands to my lap, so I wouldn't be a distraction.

"Seriously though, you know what it means?" I said. "The belt means we have four months of study behind us. Four months until the next test. It'll only get more challenging, and we have to step up our game."

• • •

36
ABOUT THAT

GRETA KNEW leaving me in a suspended state of unknowing for a long time was a key ingredient for a seizure cluster. And, fortunately, she didn't make me second-guess more than a couple days. She saw the fall on the way to work had taken its toll.

That particular night, however, was unforgettable. Well, the service was. The waitress showed once, maybe? But anyway, we settled in at iHOP, the overtly sweet all-day breakfast place.

"About what you said," she started. "It's all hard to hear."

"Yeah," I said. "About that."

"Just hear me out. I heard you out."

"You did. Sorry."

"It's hard to hear," she said. "Your angst. And probably harder to accept."

I nodded. "I knew it might be. Which was why I held it close."

She motioned for silence.

Although it always seemed full, the restaurant must have emptied or been in a lull. I hadn't seen her act so emphatically amidst a packed joint, around few contented diners for that matter.

"No excuses, here, hon," I added. "It was hard for me to express, though."

"That said," Greta spoke over me. "I did ask for it. And you gave me a lot to consider."

I nodded again.

"I mulled over it, and I get some things, but others?"

"Others," I said, finishing her thought. "You aren't so sure."

Greta sighed, then nodded.

I nervously aligned the multiple syrup containers along the back of the table. It was around then when the waitress showed once more, and offered to place them at a different table.

ELECTRIC

Just as I didn't grasp everything my dear dealt with, there were things only people with disabilities and/or Epilepsy could fathom. Would ever fathom, for that matter.

I was most eager to discover whether or not Greta could put it behind us, or if my disclosure was too much.

Would she extend the same grace I knew I had to give to Adaline?

• • •

37
MIRACLE?

I WAS DOWN to my last replacement pills. The last! I'd done everything I knew to get my hands on the needed medication. But all I got from every source was resistance.

And now I was managing the expected auras, my daily to-do list, and carrying a dark dread that perhaps it was too late, and the reality the coming week could be a traumatic one.

An under-dose could be just as bad as an overdose. I knew both all too well from accidental instances in the past. The shakiness. The headaches.

Mary Grace could traverse the Wellspan hallways all she wanted, showcasing her larger-than-life persona, but she hadn't protected me like the lioness to which I earlier compared her. Not even close.

She started out helping Rhys. And then, after facing difficulty with the insurance company, after having to answer real questions from me, it seemed she gave up. Took solace in ignorance. Well, she handed me off to the PA. A far cry from the days she was caring, the days she called me at home to see if I was hanging in there after a hard seizure.

But that's where I was at now. Home. Watching and waiting. Downing a flavored water. Drifting. Wondering again how this would all go down.

Had I missed something? Did the inability to resolve the situation on my own imply more hardship, or did it suggest a miracle was in the works?

You always hoped it was the latter.

• • •

38
OFFER

THE PRECISE timing I had to consider when consuming a meal was just one facet of the physical trigger. The content I decided on also determined the degree of coverage I could count on.

If at a given hour, I ate, for example, a high carb meal, as opposed to a high protein meal, or something sugary instead of something healthy, I not only grew tired after a brief energy spike, but I also became more prone to seize. Auras overwhelmed me.

The extended release (ER) anticonvulsants I took would last longer if they had ample roughage to slow their secretion. If not, the pills sped through my system, and didn't work. It took a lifetime of triggers, and my own observation, to arrive at this conclusion.

I was never previously attentive to my diet. Always felt if I was going to seize and hurt, I should at least have the liberty to enjoy a

TRIGGER

sweet. But since identifying potential seizure causes in content consumption, I thought about it twice.

My discovery did make me wonder one thing, though: Why hadn't the doctors—the "experts" so eager to experiment on me—ever emphasized drug effectiveness was contingent on the manner in which I ate?

• • •

WE DIDN'T unlock the deli site immediately, but my offer to do so seemed to incentivize a re-visit of and agreement on the major things: like the new brand, the color scheme, and the overall theme.

I mean, Adaline and I had already gone over so much. To address aesthetics, I just needed her to affirm my suggested direction, and let me push it to the finish line.

"Half the site is dedicated to the deli," I said. "While the other half is dedicated to your catering service."

"With the focus, I see, on the catering side."

"As you wanted."

Adaline's phone rang, but this time she didn't get up. "Will get to that later."

"The food slider on the home page really stands out."

"And we can always update that with each new season."

"The general content is much more vibrant, too."

"I agree."

I could never tell if her previous detachment had to do with self-righteousness or with disinterest. I never decided, one way or the other.

In any event, I enjoyed the new Adaline. The new improved Adaline.

• • •

39
GRIND

WHILE HANK and I took occasional breaks from class either due to inclement weather or seizure injury and/or recovery—we did our best to keep our twice-a-week practice commitment, to stick to the grind.

Life pressed on, but—to use an outdated cliché—we stuck to our guns and pressed harder. We stepped up our game.

Some weeks, it was Monday and Wednesday. Other weeks, it was Monday and Thursday. And other weeks, still, it was one day of dojo practice, and another of at-home practice.

We never went in on a weekend, although some students did. Three times a week was a lot to ask of anyone, but the idea intrigued me.

There were some instances when—right before class—I seized, and I surprised Hank with a random cancellation call or text. I felt badly when this happened. And yet, generally speaking, I didn't lose heart and was still driven to pursue the craft.

IT'S A broad statement, I know, but habits were a driving force for me. I think the same went for Hank. In the martial arts, you developed good and bad habits, and—if genuinely committed—you spent a lifetime negating the bad ones, and refining the good ones.

ELECTRIC

I'd heard one instructor say you didn't want to waste time on bad habits, but—in the context of Shotokan training—I didn't know that anything except practice would change them.

For me, I didn't technically recognize the bad habits—like over-exertion or empty punches without hip rotation or kicks without follow-through—until later in the game. But when I did, it changed everything.

At first, I was surprised, and couldn't get over how frequently and consistently each new person around me—even some who outranked me—resorted to poor form.

I saw the difference in quality, though, and I did everything in my power to achieve and sustain higher quality moves and stances.

I didn't immediately fix them all, but incrementally, one by one, I improved my flaws, enhanced my strengths, and then I passed my observations on to Hank, if he didn't notice them already.

• • •

40
ACCEPTANCE

"So I can accept you've got a history," said Greta.

"Thank you," I said. "I know it's not exclusive to me."

We sat on a bench at a city park consumed by swans. They were everywhere, the number so great their cries even drowned me out.

I wasn't really an outdoorsy type—although I walked everywhere—but it seemed a decent place to continue our chat.

"That's right," she said. "I have a history."

"About which you were candid with me."

"We all have a past. Stuff that could hang us up if we let it."

"I don't want to let it."

"Listen to me, Chris," said Greta. "I don't blame you for feeling one way or another. Although I'd prefer you only felt good about us."

"You and me both," I said. "I don't want to feel conflicted."

The kids who should have been enjoying the birds, feeding them, must have been conflicted, too, as they were obviously indoors missing out, and I'd yet to see any child around.

"I even accept your history is far more complicated than most."

I was impressed by all she was willing to accept. But, then again, I pursued her for her superior qualities.

"It's a story and a half," I agreed.

We left the park when Greta had finished her piece. And yet, despite all to which Greta had assented, she hadn't explicitly claimed everything between us was okay.

• • •

41
RACE

THERE WAS no questioning my medicine situation wasn't okay. Mary Grace ended up a more formidable foe in the race to acquire the stuff than I thought, and now a miracle was all I could trust in.

I had planned on going out around her, on leaving all impediments in the dust. But, to keep this analogy going, I couldn't propel past her. I struggled to outwit the medical establishment, and got stuck behind Mary Grace.

TRIGGER

You sometimes saw foes act as allies during a race, and—even with our past—I fully expected Mary Grace to get my back, as I didn't think she would want me to seize, regardless. But, up to this point, I was wrong.

Four thirty—closing time at the neurology clinic—came around, though, and she immediately ended her chase for the day, never crossing the finish line, never affirming I would have coverage.

• • •

42
AMOUNT

WHILE I'M still talking about the physical aspects of triggers, I should say a bit about how the amount of consumed food also impacted a day's seizure number and intensity.

All those years of college, building my life around morning, afternoon, and night time classes, I had to adapt, and grew used to eating a little here, a little there, sacrificing meals to keep a schedule, catching up with two meals worth after a four-hour (sometimes eight-hour) debate. I'd seen other students fall into the same trap. For me, though, the resulting seizures were pretty bad.

I followed a similar pattern when done with school, staying productive at a cost, living the bachelor life for what seemed an eternity, no one really there to urge me in a different direction when I wasn't hungry or preoccupied with other things.

But I didn't realize my oversight until this past year, 2016. In my 36th year, it dawned on me there was a connection between eating next to nothing around the universal eating times, and enduring a host of triggers.

There also was a connection between doing the opposite and seizures, eating a lot too late, after the excess electrical activity had already started ruling my brain.

I partially credited Greta for the understanding, but I ultimately believe—in quiet time—the Lord revealed it to me.

• • •

MENU ITEMS and meal plans: the core items—after aesthetics—Adaline wanted me to refine. They had a lot, let me tell you.

And it made sense, since their deli clientele had to choose one of many offered sandwiches, and their event clientele had to choose one of the appetizer, dinner, and dessert combos to benefit from any kind of catering.

For hours, we sat side-by-side examining the Wordpress website. How they presented the options, I soon saw, determined what dinner ingredients they would need to acquire, and what dishes they lugged around from event site to event site.

"I want the deli menu beautiful and by itself."

"Okay."

"And I want all platter choices visually pleasing, separate, and accessible."

"I can do that."

A client expressing exactly what she wanted. I'd wished for it for months, and now couldn't help but view it as a luxury.

ELECTRIC

To improve matters, I saw the years of experience (perhaps the same know-how that caused her to mistreat me, at first) in the details that sold their selection. There was a simplicity to it, and yet enough was there to imply choice and quality.

"Second to your daughter's photography," I said.

"This will be the best part of the site."

• • •

43
INTENSITY

THE OCCASIONAL breaks Hank and I took from karate practice were far and few between, but they were healthy, and, in my personal opinion, seemed to add an intensity to our efforts upon returning.

"We've got no excuse now!" I said to Hank. "A few days off to recover, we can now jump into it with a vengeance!"

I was kind of playing, but I was still pretty serious, too. I operated in this life repeatedly re-bounding and thriving after Epilepsy beat me up. How was this much different?

"Right?" I said to Hank. "Am I right?"

Hank, like usual, said, "Right." But, of late, along with his evolution as a martial artist, I felt a deeper enthusiasm and intensity from him.

Our bodies healed and our minds renewed, Hank and I quickly changed, bowed in, and then walked out onto the mats.

JOSHUA HOLMES

The class was full, and after stretching—as often seemed the case—Sensei chose the most physically challenging defense sequences to practice.

FLOOR FIGHTING—akin to yet more controlled than cage fighting—was perhaps the most exhausting, nevertheless my favorite kind of self defense.

I studied Muay Thai when I took Kali for three years in State College, too. So it was already ingrained in my head, pretty familiar to me, and I loved the challenge.

How often one relied upon or resorted to it was up for debate. That it refined your body control, split-second decision making abilities, tactile acuity, joint-manipulation skills, and guaranteed the deflection of danger was indisputable.

Back and forth, Hank and I took turns attacking from the top and bottom positions. I was in heaven, sweating up a storm, saying to my friend, "Don't hold back! Give me a run for my money!"

Hank subsequently threw some punches my way, and I had to ward them off until I had a chance to steal his arms, thrust my butt up in the air, wrap my left leg around his neck, and get him in a chokehold.

He managed to do the same to me, and considering his bulky stature, with practice, I saw him growing pretty proficient. I had to tap out when he succeeded in leg-locking me.

We went at it until we both had accrued new injuries. I could tell we both were improving more and more all the time.

• • •

TRIGGER

44
NO REASON

THERE WITH Greta, I was mentally and emotionally tired, uncertain and ready, thinking, *Well there's really no reason to draw this out any further*. For, as I mentioned, she didn't exactly say I was off the hook, but she went above and beyond to express her understanding.

I wanted to say what I would to the guys in the locker room: "So let's just cut to the chase...", but I thought better of it and edited my inquiry before voicing it.

"Can I just say your sensitivity blows me away?" I said. "And thank you again." I smiled. "I do know you well enough now, though, to see you're not finished. This is leading to your actual point."

As I hoped, Greta saw my subtle hint not to beat around the bush, and jumped at the opening.

"I'm not Mary Grace," she said. "I'm not Linda. I'm not Michael. I'm not any of the people who left you out to dry back then.

"I'm here and now. Existing. In the moment. In the present. Current.

"You don't scare me. You're condition doesn't scare me—your injuries, yes. But I'm not going anywhere.

"Unless...."

• • •

JOSHUA HOLMES

45
COLLECTION

THE PHONE ring startled me, but I automatically thought, *Could this be the call about meds?* I lifted the device from the rug to my ear on the third vibration.

I didn't recognize the number. It very well could have been a telemarketer who induced a trigger, but, fortunately, it wasn't. I assumed correctly.

"Hello Chris. It's Rhys. Can you confirm your date of birth, phone number, and address for me?"

"Hasn't the office closed?"

"Yes. But I'm still here. To get you your medicine."

She had struggled to help me, at first. Lost the responsibility, actually. And she had a kid to get home to. But she stepped up in Mary Grace's absence.

"Thank you," I said.

I went ahead and gave her the requested information.

"And you are out tonight... Am I right?"

I paced the house, back and forth. Peered through the window blinds. I then looked again at my empty pill container.

"Yeah...my backup supply is all gone," I said. "It's barely covering me as is."

"So you need both then."

I rubbed my head nervously. "Uh yeah."

"The pharmacy is open for a few more minutes," she said. "Let me get off here and call them. Will try to order you some pills."

ELECTRIC

"Okay. Thanks."

• • •

46
AVID

AN AVID coffee lover and Starbucks attendee, the final physical, trigger-oriented obstacle I still tried to understand was the almost exact fluid-to-food ratio I had to maintain.

Believe it or not, before and after a snack or meal, I had to be very conscious about the quantity of liquid I drank.

For, if my coffee (tea or water) intake exceeded my meal amount, it likely would diminish my anti-convulsants' potency, if not entirely nullify their purpose.

Alternately, if I deprived myself of adequate fluids, the suggested six cups, I could easily get dehydrated, quickly leading to triggers, as well.

I wasn't a dietitian or food expert, by any means, and the balancing act was exactly that: arduous trial and error, possible to carry out, but equally prone to mistakes; experimentation that continued beyond the neurology clinic.

One might read this and conclude, in order to thrive with Epilepsy, you had to pay the above areas their demanded attention and take the required steps. I would agree. I continue to give the issues notice. And yet there is nothing easy or natural about it

• • •

JOSHUA HOLMES

THE WEB development process with Adaline—after assembling lists of menu options and meal choices—did, however, start progressing with ease and begin feeling more natural. I still wondered how it was possible, as it required a major attitudinal shift.

With that—upon seeing adjustments as a regular part of website creation, and, given the opportunity, they were a breeze for me to accomplish—Adaline continued to adjust and grow more direct.

Each freelance project had its highs and lows, its interpersonal demands, its joys and frustrations—perhaps a few extra for me due to my approach (depending who you asked)—and yet, when all was said and done, the majority of my projects ended successfully.

Adaline and everyone at The Festive Shore were a classic case; One that started a mess, and one that managed to come around.

I walked away with the rest of my money, the winner of a prizefight, and they walked away with an improved brand and web presence.

• • •

47
STATE OF MIND

HANK AND I stood side by side, watching Sensei teach us across the room, look everyone in the eye, point at his head, and say, "Ladies and gentlemen, more than anything, it all starts here." He tapped the side of his skull again. "Right here."

Most of us shouted in acknowledgment.

"Now who can tell me what that means?"

TRIGGER

Sensei had always encouraged everyone to speak up, but emphasized the importance of confidently owning what you said, ignorant or otherwise.

So one of the fearless youngsters offered a possible meaning.

"Okay, that's good," said Sensei. "What I mean, though, guys, is the martial arts is a state of mind. Self-defense is a state of mind."

I felt I'd talked to Hank about this very thing a million times; How you could see the natural fighter vs. the learned fighter; How it all returned to the mental stance one had.

"Are you going to be the one who defeats, or the one who is defeated?"

The curtains were drawn, the punching bags were stacked, and we were instructed to find an open wall.

I turned to Hank and asked if he felt he could go to the "aggressor mind space", for lack of a better term, when he practiced with me, and he looked back at me and said, "You know? I think I can."

The next test was weeks away, and Hank's skillset was getting better all the time. He took me down well that night.

I noticed a positive shift in Hank's mindset, in his fighting style. It thrilled me, and felt like a victory in its own right.

The speech validated what I already believed to be true. I fought to defeat, no matter what, all the time, even amidst the unknown.

• • •

48
FORGIVEN

"UNLESS," I interrupted Greta. "I stay in the past. I get it."

It wasn't a surprise expectation: to live in the present. Nor was it unreasonable. It was, however, one a long time coming.

"You do," she said, as if to confirm.

"I understand," I said. "Honestly. Already moving on."

"Moving on," repeated Greta.

"So you forgive me, then?"

I knew my question might convey flippancy (though it wasn't my intent), and anticipated a pause or a breath. But Greta surprised me with an immediate answer, followed by a kiss.

"I forgive you."

I reached for her hand, which was soft yet secure in mine, lifted her to her feet, and said, "Let's go home. I've had my fill of dinners out."

"Yeah. Me too."

• • •

49
LATE

I NEVER HEARD back from Rhys regarding my meds, but I was startled one last time pretty late that evening, as an elderly man pounded on my front door.

An hour passed after my talk with Rhys, and I continued to wait and see—again in a suspended state—how it all would unfold. I was at the mercy of a purple-haired, young girl with good intentions and a pharmacist with an open heart.

I couldn't believe how close they'd cut it, but was relieved to discover the older gentleman at the door was the delivery guy.

ELECTRIC

"Hello young man," said the delivery guy. "Please sign here."

I went ahead and signed the receipt, and took the bag of meds.

I felt as if I'd been on a roller coaster, had endured the slowest, extraordinary climb to the ride's peak, and plummeted straight down when the track fell away from beneath me. And yet, somehow, in the end I sat there with my medicine in my lap, protected last minute.

I shook my head and took the new containers back to the restroom.

• • •

EPILOGUE
GRATIFIED

IT WAS gratifying, weeks later, to see those closest to me—Greta, Foster, even Adaline—venture out in the late evening to support me, to arrive at the secluded dojo, and enter to observe Hank and me practice and spar.

It was equally pleasing to see absolutely no sign of Mary Grace or any other POCAs. For at least one enjoyable session, my medical issues, and those loosely connected, would keep a distance.

"You made it," I said. "Awesome."

"Wouldn't miss it," said Foster. "Not when home from a trip."

"Thanks for the invite," said Adaline.

"A treat," I said. "A real treat to have you."

I smiled at my other observers, waved, and then returned to the demonstration in progress. Eager, I suppose, because I was ready to compete.

JOSHUA HOLMES

I could now focus on watching my opponent, on dancing around, and on landing some blows, because, last minute, my biggest distraction—the medicine—was dropped off at my house, which gave me another month to sort things out. And the lady of the hour, Greta, put to rest my second distraction—her potential departure.

Sensei stopped demonstrating; looked at me, and then looked at Rahal; called us out onto the floor; instructed us to bow to each other, and to bow to him.

Per his instruction, I went out there adorned in bright red gear, and, with heart, fought the highest rank I had to date, in a way unique to me. I was hardly crisp, and yet I was quick and aggressive, fearless, and determined.

"Relax," said Sensei. "Just relax."

I breathed deeply, continued to circle, and went back into it.

Greta laughed from her seat, giddy when I managed to knock down a block and connect a punch. "Nice work, Chris!"

One peer offered, "Beautiful block!"

"Right there," Another said. "Give him a combo!"

A few more minutes, I defended myself well. Following the punch, I thrust a couple kicks; snapped Rahal's gut once.

And just as quickly as Sensei started the spar, he called it to a close. We all bowed again out of respect.

"Strong performance, Chris," said Rahal.

"I agree," said Sensei.

"I felt good about it."

"Right," said Hank, who would also have a good showing.

TRIGGER

"That was really great," added Rahal. "Now to get your legs as fast as your hands."

It was great. And it would continue to be.

"Yeah," I said. "Like trigger-fast."

• • •

ACKNOWLEDGMENTS

Thanks to God, my Parents, and Grandparents

ACKNOWLEDGMENTS

Thanks to God, my Parents, and Grandparents

www.ingramcontent.com/pod-product-compliance
Lightning Source LLC
Chambersburg PA
CBHW052236220526
45471CB00001B/65